"Dr. Byock's book rejuvenates me professionally. In allowing us the special privilege of entering the sacred space of their final journey, people teach us precious lessons about ourselves. Dr. Byock has a gift of sharing the lessons he's learned in a most readable narrative marked by compassion, love of life, and lucidity."

—*Rabbi Bunny Freedman, founding director, Jewish Hospice & Chaplaincy Network*

"In *The Best Care Possible*, Ira Byock tells us why we need to move beyond medicine's fixation on conquering death to a vision of end-of-life care focused on the quality of the patient's experience. This is a beautifully written, highly personal account that makes real the struggle of patients and families to escape the "high-tech," more-is-better imperative that dominates the American way of death. It provides compelling examples of how the physician, committed to reform, can help patients achieve the care they want and need. But Byock goes further: he makes the case that professional reform is only part of the solution; overcoming the medicalization of death will require the mobilization of the wider community in the support of the dying (and those with chronic illness)."

— *Jack Wennberg, M.D., author of* Tracking Medicine:
A Researcher's Quest to Understand Health Care

"Once again, Dr. Ira Byock delivers a message of hope and promise to all of us who will face our own deaths. Dying is always sad, but with proper professional insight and skill an individual's last chapter need not be dominated by suffering and isolation. Dr. Byock demonstrates that growth and completion are possible in the midst of grief and loss. His clinical stories and commentary point to the resilience people find and the importance they discover in their relationships as they face life's final challenges. This is an important look at the personal, social, and political implications of how we care for one another and how we die. *The Best Care Possible* is a rallying cry to all of us who are concerned about the direction of health care in the United States."

—*Donald Schumacher, Psy.D., president and CEO, National Hospice and Palliative Care Organization*

"Having traveled this landscape with loved ones, taking care of individuals at the end of their life is both a privilege and a tremendous challenge, both physically and spiritually. We need a map. Ira Byock has created a map of compassionate intelligence for palliative care with grace. Through the power of story and his own intuitive sense of what dignity means to the dying, this is more than a manual; it is a godsend. It is also a call for health care with heart, conscience, and consequences."

—*Terry Tempest Williams, author of* Refuge

The Best
Care Possible

The Best Care Possible

A Physician's Quest to Transform Care

Through the End of Life

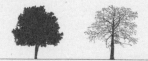

IRA BYOCK, M.D.

AVERY

a member of Penguin Group (USA) Inc.

New York

Published by the Penguin Group
Penguin Group (USA) Inc., 375 Hudson Street, New York, New York 10014,
USA • Penguin Group (Canada), 90 Eglinton Avenue East, Suite 700, Toronto, Ontario
M4P 2Y3, Canada (a division of Pearson Penguin Canada Inc.) • Penguin Books Ltd,
80 Strand, London WC2R 0RL, England • Penguin Ireland, 25 St Stephen's Green,
Dublin 2, Ireland (a division of Penguin Books Ltd) • Penguin Group (Australia),
250 Camberwell Road, Camberwell, Victoria 3124, Australia (a division of Pearson Australia
Group Pty Ltd) • Penguin Books India Pvt Ltd, 11 Community Centre, Panchsheel Park,
New Delhi–110 017, India • Penguin Group (NZ), 67 Apollo Drive, Rosedale, North
Shore 0632, New Zealand (a division of Pearson New Zealand Ltd) • Penguin Books
(South Africa) (Pty) Ltd, 24 Sturdee Avenue, Rosebank, Johannesburg 2196, South Africa

Penguin Books Ltd, Registered Offices: 80 Strand, London WC2R 0RL, England

Most Avery books are available at special quantity discounts for bulk purchase for
sales promotions, premiums, fund-raising, and educational needs. Special books or
book excerpts also can be created to fit specific needs. For details, write Penguin
Group (USA) Inc. Special Markets, 375 Hudson Street, New York, NY 10014.

Library of Congress Cataloging-in-Publication Data
Byock, Ira.
The best care possible: a physician's quest to transform care through the end of life / Ira Byock.
p.   cm.
ISBN 978-1-58333-459-1
I. Title.
[DNLM: 1. Palliative Care—United States.   2. Terminal Care—United States.   3. Attitude to
Death—United States.   4. Quality of Life—United States, WB 310]
2011047587
616.02'9—dc23

Printed in the United States of America
1   3   5   7   9   10   8   6   4   2

BOOK DESIGN BY NICOLE LAROCHE

ALWAYS LEARNING   PEARSON

To Yvonne

Author's Note

This book is not intended to be reportage. I have written from my personal and professional experience and the experiences of people I have met through my clinical work. A number of stories are accounts of actual persons, told as faithfully as I am able. In most instances, I have changed identifying details and people's names to preserve their privacy. Some people's real names appear in the Acknowledgments. Other stories are composites drawn from two or more patients and families I have known.

In general, the situations and conversations are reconstructions from my memory and any contemporaneous notes and quotes. In writing several stories, I complemented my contemporaneous notes with subsequent interviews with patients, family members, and clinicians.

The subtitle, *A Physician's Quest to Transform Care Through the End of Life*, is intended to set this book in the first person. This is my perspective. I do not represent or speak for any organization or group. However, this quest is not exclusive. People from a variety of disciplines and walks of life are working to transform care for people through the end of life. Over several decades many physicians, nurses, and other health care professionals have contributed to developing the field of hospice and palliative care. I feel privileged to count myself among them.

Contents

Introduction

Americans are scared to death of dying. And with good reason. While rarely easy under any circumstances, we make dying a lot harder than it has to be.

A large majority of Americans still die in hospitals or nursing homes. Many suffer poorly controlled pain or other physical miseries and endure their final days feeling undignified and a burden to others.

Few of us can even imagine how things might be different. Therein lies the crux of the problem. Our society and mainstream American culture have never grappled with the fundamental fact of mortality; therefore, we do not know what to expect or what is possible. When someone we love is diagnosed with a life-threatening condition, the worst thing we can imagine is that he or she might die. The sobering fact is that there are worse things than having someone you love die. Most basic, there is having the person you love die badly, suffering as he or she dies. Worse still is realizing later on that much of his or her suffering was unnecessary.

This book is about understanding the dangers that confront seriously ill and dying people and their families, and avoiding the pitfalls that

ensnare so many. It is about how things could be better—much better—
for ourselves, the people we love, and, eventually, for our national community and culture. Most immediately, *The Best Care Possible* is about
how to make the best of what is often the very worst time of life.

When it comes to caring for people with advanced illnesses, our
social systems are so broken and our health care system is so dysfunctional and, frankly, neglectful that it would be easy to become furious. In
truth, however, this predicament is no one's fault. It is a consequence of
living in remarkable, unprecedented times.

Death is the most inevitable fact of life. But the experience of dying
has changed over the course of history, especially within the past fifty
years. In many ways dying has become a lot harder. We are the bene-
factors and victims of scientific success. Serious, chronic illness is an
invention of the late twentieth century, the fruit of our species' intel-
lectual prowess, the culmination (at least so far) of millennia of scientific progress. Throughout history, Homo sapiens have mostly died
quickly. Primitives commonly died in childbirth or as infants. Children
and adults died due to trauma and infections that today would be considered almost trivial, things like appendicitis or a fall that results in an
open arm bone fracture that then gets infected. But our ancestors also
died in short order from cancer, kidney failure, and heart failure, which
people in the twenty-first century are either cured of or live with for
many months or years.

These advances exemplify the good fortune we have to be living in
the present day. But our species' epochal success in staving off death
impacts contemporary individual and communal life in ways we have
yet to understand. Prolonged serious illness, physical dependence,
senescence, and senility are now common facts of late life. Our society
and culture—all of our respective cultures—must factor this new normal "waning stage of life" into our expectations and plans.

It is not easy to die well in modern times.

Because so many treatments now work, many people survive longer with one, or several, previously lethal conditions. Clinicians now talk about a patient's "illness burden," a term for the accumulated aches, pains, and disabilities that come with diseases and the side effects of treatment. As odd as it may sound, people are sicker before they die today than ever before.

In general, our health care system doesn't do a good job of helping people deal with the burden of illness. Striking medical advances in prolonging or replacing organ functions have not been matched by proficiency in preserving comfort and quality of life for people who are ill or their families. Even in otherwise excellent medical centers, conscientious professionals lack key skills that are essential for comprehensive caring. Busy clinicians tend to give short shrift to communicating fully with patients, treating pain or nausea or difficulty sleeping, or coordinating appointments for blood and imaging tests, office visits, medications, and transmitting critical information among various specialists. The unwavering focus on treatments for sustaining life can leave someone who is living with an advanced disease physically uncomfortable, feeling lost and confused, not knowing how to get through each day or how to plan for the future.

Nearly everyone who is asked where they would want to spend their final days says at home, surrounded by people they know and love and who love them. That's the consistent finding of public opinion surveys and, in my experience as a doctor, remains true when people become patients. Unfortunately, it is not the way things turn out. At present, just over one-fifth of Americans are at home when they die. Instead, over 30 percent die in nursing homes, where, according to opinion polls, virtually no one says they want to be. Hospitals remain the site of over 50 percent of deaths in most parts of the country, and nearly 40 percent of people who die in a hospital spend their last days in an ICU (intensive care unit), where they will likely be sedated or have their arms tied down so they will not pull out breathing tubes, intravenous lines, or catheters.

Dying is hard, but it does not have to be *this hard*.

As the process of dying has changed, so, too, caregiving has become much harder than it used to be. Modern civilization's historic successes against disease have multiplied both the complexity and duration of family caregiving. Today, more than 60 million Americans are tending a frail elder or sick child or adult at home. Even otherwise excellent medical treatments and hospital care may leave a family not knowing how to care well at home for a dying loved one. By the end of a long illness, family caregivers are commonly physically and emotionally exhausted. Up to a third of close family members of people treated in an ICU experience anxiety or depression consistent with post-traumatic stress disorder. In a health surveillance study, family caregivers who reported the highest levels of emotional or physical strain from caregiving had nearly two-thirds higher risk of dying in a four-year period than age-matched controls.

Caregiving is hard, but it does not have to be *this hard*.

Clearly, a transformation is needed in the way our society and culture—not merely our health care system—cares for seriously ill people and supports family caregivers.

Right now, effective advocacy by patients and families is needed to avoid common mistakes, avert suffering, and prevent regrets. Knowing what to expect, what to demand, and what limitations to accept can lessen the burdens of illness and caregiving.

The collective impact of longer lives and common periods of physical dependency affect the economic well-being of individuals, families, and society as a whole. Families commonly miss the lost income that results from sickness and caregiving, absorb out-of-pocket expenses, and worry that costs might exceed the lifetime limits of insurance coverage. Tens of thousands of home foreclosures are attributable to lost wages and medical costs of long-term illnesses. Even before the recent deep, prolonged recession, well over a million American families annually filed for bankruptcy due to health care costs. Aggregate health care expenses are felt by employers, large and small, and by all of us who pay taxes that underwrite Medicare and Medicaid. These medical costs erode our national capacity to engage in other pressing priorities: education, social services, and our country's infrastructure of bridges, roads, railways, and information highways.

As difficult as things are now, these may turn out to be the good old days. How we die is already a public health crisis, and care for people through the end of life is poised to become a generation-long social catastrophe. Within the next few years, a demographic tidal wave of aging and chronically ill Americans will overwhelm our already stressed systems. As a nation, time is fleeting to avert a full-blown disaster.

Very soon, for the first time in human history, older people will outnumber younger people on our planet. In the United States, one in five adults is sixty-five or older. The 75 million baby boomers have begun paying senior prices at the box office and every day thousands more qualify for Medicare and Social Security. Consider that in 1940, when Social Security benefits were first paid, there were an estimated 41 workers paying into the fund for every recipient of benefits. This ratio has progressively diminished and is on track to be 2.1 workers for every beneficiary by 2030. Those of us who are concerned about long-term care have good reasons to worry. The nursing homes of the future—*our future!*—may make today's nursing homes look like luxury hotels.

It doesn't have to turn out that way.

Living in unprecedented times is not all bad. Quite the contrary: the historic challenges we face come with historic opportunities. As a society, we can collectively transform the way we die. But if we want to reclaim a sense of optimism about our future—and our children's futures—we must act wisely, courageously, and decisively.

As important as doing something is, before leaping into action, it is worth pausing to understand why we haven't taken action sooner. I am not the first person to note that our nation's social systems and services have not kept pace with advances in treatments and survival, leaving urgent catch-up work to be done. For years sociologists, public health professionals, gerontologists, and members of my own field of palliative care have been warning about the looming problems of aging, dying, and caregiving. In 1997 the Institute of Medicine concluded, "Too many people suffer needlessly at the end of life, both from errors of omission and commission." One reason our nation hasn't acted sooner is that there are always more immediate crises to deal with: terrorism, foreign wars, hurricanes, floods, the bursting of financial bubbles, and the near collapse of our economy. All rightly vie for attention of the voting public, politicians, and elected leaders. However, competing social priorities alone do not explain our country's inaction on these pressing issues.

Let's face it: A more basic reason is that the subject of how we die is depressing. *"I don't want to think about it!"* aptly expresses the American mind-set. Our cultural tendency is to avoid serious conversations about the end of life. Pain, pus, puking, being at the mercy of doctors, the astronomical expenses, the utter disruption of life. Who wants to think about any of that?

The complex social and system challenges we face make it all the more tempting for politicians and social leaders to keep deflecting—or at least deferring—the topic. Public policy discussions related to incurable illness, dying, death, and grief are typically confined to either the costs of health care or the pros and cons of physician-assisted suicide. Neither are adequate proxies for the fundamental questions of how our society should respond to our most fragile elderly or ill members and the families who care for them. Politicians shy away from the issues because they don't want to depress voters. Savvy candidates strive to ignite a sense of optimism and can-do enthusiasm among voters—even if doing so means postponing some pressing social responsibilities. The topic of how we die is just not energizing.

And, of course, as mentioned, there are always more urgent problems to attend to, which provide plausible cover for putting off these morbid discussions. So, like passengers on a river raft we drift along, toward a precipice we have been told lies ahead, effectively distracted and seemingly unaware that the longer we wait, the harder it will be to avoid disaster.

Last, and most maddening, mortality has recently become a politically polarized issue. It is almost comical, but the consequences aren't funny. One would think that mortality would provide the ultimate common ground for bringing people together. Instead, suspicion pervades and divides public opinion on the way we die. In addition to being depressing, the subject has now become politically toxic.

On the one hand, ardent proponents of legalizing physician-assisted suicide accuse doctors of forcing people to suffer by refusing to prescribe lethal medications. Doctors and nurses who do not support right-to-die legislation are alleged to hide a religious agenda or have a profit motive in keeping patients alive.

On the other hand, vehement elements of the Pro-life movement accuse doctors and nurses of promoting "a culture of death" whenever we allow people to die gently—without subjecting them to CPR (cardiopulmonary resuscitation), breathing machines, dialysis, or feeding tubes. Vocal Pro-lifers loudly equate writing a DNR (do not resuscitate) order with killing patients, advance care planning conversations between doctors and patients with "death panels," and palliative care with rationing or "killing granny."

The only thing these two passionate and disparate poles of public opinion have in common is a deep-seated distrust of doctors and nurses, the very professionals society relies on at the end of life.

No wonder our politicians and elected officials avoid these topics as if they were radioactive. Year after year, pressing problems that deserve—and might be solved by—thoughtful consideration and constructive public policy remain unattended. Needless suffering continues. This seems the very definition of social irresponsibility. Fixable problems go unfixed and far too many Americans die badly. No wonder there is public distrust.

What a morass.

Unless and until we can bridge the cultural chasm of distrust, we will not substantially improve the way we die.

Most practitioners in my own field of hospice and palliative care largely choose to ignore the outrageous allegations that we promote death panels and the killing of vulnerable people. In being too polite, or too timid, to confront the controversy, I fear that we have allowed the distrust to fester. To a public that is worried about care, silence from the accused can be easily misconstrued. Uncorrected accusations reverberate within media echo chambers. Unchecked, political vitriol of this nature will derail socially responsible, constructive actions. It's unnecessary.

In truth, reverence for life permeates the care that I and colleagues in our field provide. Love for life motivates everything that I do and teach. Reverence for life does not include hastening death, nor does it include forcing people to suffer as they die. As a clinician, it does require me to show up—with all the resources and skills my training and experience provide—and to lean forward, listening to the persons before me and learning how I can best be of service.

I don't think of myself as religious. I was raised by Jewish parents, and although I am not particularly observant of holidays or rituals, my sense of the inherent value of life has roots deep within my ancestry and upbringing. Life is an absolute value for Jews. Many Jews wear the Hebrew symbol for life, *chai*, as pendants around their necks. We toast *L'chaim!* (To life!) as we raise glasses in celebration. If reverence for life constitutes a religious agenda, I suppose I have one.

However, the value of life is embedded in secular medical and nursing care as well. It is also, of course, evident in health care chaplaincy, regardless of the individual chaplain's faith. Life's intrinsic value motivates clinical trainees and professionals of every discipline. Although many of the patients we care for could be considered to be dying, my experience of hospice and palliative care is of an unrestrained team effort to preserve, honor, and celebrate life.

The branding of the term "Pro-life" by conservative political activists has had an unhelpful, polarizing effect on the culture. People who are not "Pro-life" are, therefore, what? Pro-death? I don't think so.

In truth, my colleagues and I in hospice and palliative care represent the most genuinely Pro-life segment of American society. An unwavering affirmation of life leads most of us to oppose legalizing assisted suicide and euthanasia. But it is not about politics. It is simply that love of life—not in the abstract but love for the people we care for as patients— is the reason we do what we do. People who work in this field understand that to truly affirm life, one needs to affirm *all* of life—and that includes the part that we call "dying."

An authentic, consistent Pro-life message could resolve cultural controversies surrounding how we die. Knowing that, in addition to alleviating symptoms and distress, we can honor and celebrate the people we love as they die opens up fresh approaches to difficult, unavoidable life-and-death decisions. The ethics of care must no longer be confined to considerations of when and under what circumstances life-prolonging treatments can be withheld or withdrawn. Ethics must elaborate when and under what circumstances we must act to enhance a person's comfort, sense of dignity, and well-being through the end of life.

I am convinced that Americans across the social and political spectrum can come to broad agreement on what the best care possible looks like and what it means to die well. Most people already agree on the fundamentals of high-quality care. We can stand on common ground well above the scarred fields of old culture wars. We can provide excellent lifesaving treatments, while respecting people's right to determine when enough is enough, always ensuring that their pain is treated expertly, that they and their families are treated tenderly.

Sadly, the way many Americans die remains a national disgrace. Yet, this is one national crisis we can solve. To succeed we must face hard truths and act courageously. We must be willing to collaborate even when—*especially when*—our social, religious, and political beliefs and personal preferences are very different. The stories that fill *The Best Care Possible* are evidence that medical excellence and tender human caring can coexist.

Upon closing this book, I hope you will have a sense of what "the best care possible" looks like in the twenty-first century. And if a time comes when you need it, I hope you will be prepared to get the very best care for you and those you love.

Part One

The Best
Care Possible

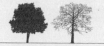

The Best Care Possible

Gerry Thorsen sat across from me in the examination room, next to his wife, Elaine. He did not look ill, far from it. He appeared healthy and considerably younger than his seventy-two years. I glanced at his date of birth on the identification stickers of his chart's billing sheet; it confirmed his age. His pink cheeks and tanned, deeply freckled scalp were noticeable during our overcast late fall in New England. His lean, muscular frame filled the arms and chest of a gray turtleneck, beneath the blue polar fleece vest he wore. I thought to myself that Mr. Thorsen had the look of a veteran distance runner—someone who might be profiled in *Parade*, a senior health magazine, or AARP's *Bulletin*.

I was glad he appeared so well, but I knew that he was seriously ill.

At the moment, Gerry Thorsen also looked like someone who was feeling vulnerable and a bit bewildered. I introduced myself as a physician from the Palliative Care Service, quickly adding that our team focuses on people's comfort and quality of life, and that it is routine at this cancer center for us to see patients recently diagnosed with pancreatic cancer. I explained that our team often helps people through treatments in ways that are medical—such as helping to manage side effects of treatments—but also practical and personal.

His face relaxed. "Oh, that sounds good. To be honest, we were not sure why we were here. We were given this appointment but didn't know what palliative care was. We looked it up on the Web and it said it had something to do with hospice. But I am not ready for that."

Until a few weeks ago, as far as he knew, Gerry Thorsen had been in peak health. I commented that he looked fit and asked if he exercised regularly. He explained that he usually exercises every day, either outdoors or, if the weather is really bad, at a fitness club. He gave up marathons six years ago when he had his right knee replacement, but he still plays tennis, jogs, bicycles, or, in the winter, cross-country skis most days.

"At least I did," he said. His voice trailed off and he gazed at the floor as he paused. He looked at me before continuing.

He said that he and Elaine, also in her early seventies, often hiked together three seasons of the year and skied together each winter. I asked if he had a connection with Killington, the Vermont ski area whose logo was embroidered on the left breast of his vest.

"I have been on the ski patrol there for fifteen years," he said, adding, "I guess this year may be an exception."

Since retiring from his own real estate business seven years ago, the Thorsens have traveled at least eight or ten weeks each year—mostly to Chicago and San Francisco, where their son and daughter live, with their spouses and the Thorsens' young grandchildren. They had also taken walking tours in England, Ireland, Italy, and the Himalayas.

"We have a good life," he concluded.

A week before Halloween their life changed. Gerry began having pain in the pit of his stomach that ached into his back. He cast it off as indigestion, took Prilosec OTC each morning and a laxative every other day. Occasionally, for a few hours at a time, he felt better. After two weeks, however, the pain was more constant and he decided to see

Grant Edwards, his family doctor. An examination and routine blood tests showed that his serum bilirubin and alkaline phosphatase, two tests of liver function, were elevated. An ultrasound scan of his abdomen, performed at their local hospital, showed that the bile ducts in his liver were enlarged. Even though no gallstones were seen on the ultrasound, the most common cause of these symptoms remained small stones or sludge from the gallbladder blocking the bile ducts. The next morning, a gastroenterologist placed a fiber-optic scope through his mouth and throat, traversed his stomach, and looked at the ampulla, or opening, of the common bile duct and pancreatic duct as they drain into the duodenum. He placed an 8-millimeter tube or stent through the opening, releasing a small gush of thick bile and pus. The gastroenterologist administered one dose of an intravenous antibiotic to prevent an infection from the procedure and sent Mr. Thorsen home on oral antibiotics three times a day. The pain disappeared. Over the weekend, he felt great.

On Monday afternoon, Grant Edwards's office manager called to say that the doctor wanted Mr. Thorsen and his wife to come to his office at five p.m. "This can't be good," Gerry said to Elaine. It was 5:35 before Dr. Edwards finally was free and able to sit with the couple. He explained that the brushings of cells that the gastroenterologist had taken from the blocked bile ducts were positive for pancreatic cancer. He said plainly that this was a very serious diagnosis and that this type of cancer was definitely life threatening. Dr. Edwards told them that there were treatments available and that because his cancer was found early, there was a chance that it was curable. He referred him to Dr. Marc Pipas, the head of the pancreatic cancer program at Dartmouth-Hitchcock Medical Center's (DHMC) Norris Cotton Cancer Center.

That was just two and a half weeks before our visit.

"It all seems so sudden," Mr. Thorsen said.

Since that Monday afternoon, Mr. Thorsen underwent a CT (computerized tomography) scan to reveal the exact anatomy of his tumor and the extent to which it invaded other tissues or enclosed the major arteries and veins of the stomach, liver, and small intestine. His case was discussed at GI Tumor Board, a weekly meeting in which specialists in medical, surgical, and radiation treatment of cancer, along with palliative care specialists, dieticians, and physical therapists discuss the optimal treatments for each patient's specific condition. The consensus of the Tumor Board was for Gerry Thorsen to continue the staging evaluation and, if no spread of the cancer was found, to recommend aggressive, potentially curative treatment.

Six days later, he underwent a diagnostic laparoscopy, an outpatient operation. Under general anesthesia, a surgeon made an incision above his umbilicus, inserted a scope into his abdomen, and looked for any signs of cancer deposits on and around the liver that were too small to be seen on CT scans or MRIs (magnetic resonance imagings). Fortunately, none were found. That meant that Mr. Thorsen was eligible for neoadjuvant treatment—a combination of chemotherapy followed by radiation treatments—designed to shrink the tumor in preparation for surgery to remove it all. It is an arduous course of treatment, but the surgery—the Whipple procedure in which most or all of the pancreas, part of the stomach, the duodenum (first portion of the small intestine), and the common bile duct are removed and new passages for the flow of bile and food are created—remains the only chance people with pancreatic cancer have of being cured.

And it is a slim enough chance at that. There is roughly a 75 percent chance of getting through neoadjuvant treatment and having surgery. Even after this radical surgery, chances of being alive at five years are just over 20 percent. But without undergoing a Whipple, the chance is nil.

Pancreatic cancer is diagnosed in nearly forty-five thousand Americans every year. Men and women are equally at risk. It is the tenth most common cancer but the fourth leading cause of cancer deaths. By the time cancer of the pancreas is detected, it has often spread beyond the pancreas to encase blood vessels, track along small nerves, or seed lymph nodes. All too commonly when it is diagnosed, cancer cells have spread beyond the pancreas, invading the duodenum or sending satellite tumors into the liver or beyond. Although nearly 25 percent of people diagnosed with pancreatic cancer are alive in one year, barely 6 percent are still alive at five years. With rare exceptions, all who survive have undergone a Whipple operation. The chance of curing even one in twenty people diagnosed with pancreatic cancer fuels the hopes of patients and doctors alike. Medical oncologists and cancer surgeons typically remember the names and faces of every patient with pancreatic cancer they have cured.

One very public example of success appears to be Supreme Court Justice Ruth Bader Ginsburg whose pancreatic cancer was found at a very early stage. Early in 2009 she had a CT scan performed for routine follow-up on colon cancer for which she had undergone surgery, chemotherapy, and radiation treatments a decade earlier. Justice Ginsburg underwent a Whipple procedure in February 2009 and, as far as we know, remains free of pancreatic cancer today.

The potential for pushing the envelope of cure and of long-term survival of people with this disease motivated me to become active in the multidisciplinary pancreatic cancer team at Dartmouth, which conducts research on new treatments. Therefore, I was familiar with the sequence of procedures the Thorsens described. Indeed, things were proceeding according to a well worked out plan. The Dartmouth clinical research group designed this sequence of diagnostic and staging tests to minimize time between the diagnosis of pancreatic cancer and initiation of treatment. Cancer biology mandates haste: delays decrease chances for cure. So time is of the essence.

Gerry and Elaine Thorsen, however, felt as though they had stepped on a moving walkway, which quickly accelerated to a breathtaking speed, compelling them to hold on for dear life. They were composed as we discussed his health and upcoming treatments, but I could almost hear a whoosh in the ether surrounding them. I knew the pace was probably in his best interest; still, they looked like they could use a breather.

Doctors are often criticized for becoming callous to patients' feelings. In trying to remain sensitive to what patients may be experiencing, one simple practice I have is to ask myself how I would feel in similar circumstances. Even now, after thirty-four years of clinical practice, much of it in hospice and palliative care, when I think of being diagnosed with cancer, I imagine taking a few weeks to get away. My fantasy is to go to a beach somewhere—to take stock, get some perspective, consider my choices, and rest before starting treatments. The rational part of me fully realizes how unlikely it is that I would have the chance. The fantasy persists because it is hard to imagine being sucked so abruptly into the diagnosis and treatment vortex.

In reality, when someone is diagnosed with a serious illness, such as cancer, or a dangerous, progressive heart, lung, kidney, liver, or neurological condition, most often the disease imposes its own agenda. In order to get the best care, it is usually necessary to start right way. There are almost always more tests needed in order to determine which potential treatments would be best so that the person can make an informed decision. Even if the condition is changing slowly, these illnesses are so scary that people naturally feel pressure to do something.

The Thorsens certainly did. Less than three weeks after Gerry Thorsen went to see Dr. Edwards for a stomachache, here we were, on a Thursday afternoon in November, one week before Thanksgiving, in a small unadorned exam room at Dartmouth-Hitchcock's Norris Cotton Cancer Center in Lebanon, New Hampshire.

They had driven an hour and a quarter from central Vermont, parked, registered for the day, and had just come from the lab where he had his blood drawn. He had just seen Dr. Pipas and, after our visit, he would be headed to the infusion suite to begin chemotherapy. I was hustling to stay on time and not keep the Thorsens waiting; I had just printed, signed, and delivered three prescriptions and said good-bye to the previous patient on my morning schedule.

From reviewing his medical chart earlier that morning, I knew the basics of Gerry Thorsen's medical history, the recent diagnostic and staging scans and tests he'd been through, and the current plan for treating his cancer. I also knew his age and that the couple had been married for thirty-two years. Yet on entering the room, I'd been surprised by how young and fit they both seemed. Meeting them socially, I probably would have guessed they were in their early sixties.

Seeing him appear so healthy, and recognizing how threatened his life was, reminded me to consciously take a breath and slow down. I smiled in greeting and let a moment of silence—probably all of two or three seconds—pass as I deliberately changed pace. I was acutely aware that this normal workday morning for me was part of a surreal, shattering, and life-changing experience for the couple before me.

Gerry asked me to tell them more about palliative care and what our team could do for them.

"Simply put, our job is to make sure you and your family receive the best care possible." I chose my words carefully. I explained that cancer affects more than a person's physical health. It is well-recognized that being diagnosed with cancer affects how people feel, and not just physically. It affects their plans, their jobs, their hopes and fears for the future. It changes things overnight.

"Amen to that," he said, nodding.

"To state an obvious fact," I said, "I learned a long time ago that when one person gets a diagnosis, their family gets an illness." I paused. His expression was serious but attentive. "That is nobody's fault," I continued. "It is just part of human nature. It is because we love one another."

He turned from me to his wife and as their eyes met, they half smiled and tears welled in his eyes. He barely blinked and made no motion to wipe them.

"This has been like being kicked in the head by a mule," he said. "I served in the army for three years, half of the time in Vietnam. I promised myself that if I got home in one piece, I would never complain about anything again. And I kept that promise."

He said that through all of his years, whatever his problems at work, difficulties with personal finances, even through the deaths of his and Elaine's parents and two brothers, he had been a "glass half full" kind of a guy. Now, however, he was having a hard time staying positive.

Elaine had been quiet, appearing to be consumed with thought, occasionally nodding her head in agreement. Now she spoke up. "It's true. 'Kicked in the head by a mule' is what our daughter—who is a writer—called it on a blog she started. Gerry has always been the most upbeat person I know. But it has been hard trying to stay upbeat with what we've been reading about this cancer. It is all so unreal."

It is remarkable how often people mention a sense of unreality in talking about recent diagnoses and the impact on their lives. "This can't be happening," people plaintively declare. But of course, it can happen. For the Thorsens it was happening.

"This is hard. There is no getting around it," I said. "As I think you have been told, the treatments that lie ahead are no picnic. There is no way to sugarcoat the situation. All I can say is that we will all do whatever we can to support you both through it. We all work closely together around here—the medical oncologists, surgeons, radiation treatment specialists, and our team in palliative care. We all agree that in addition to fighting this cancer, your well-being matters. That is our palliative care team's special focus."

I paused. Despite the weight of all we had discussed, the mood in the room was lighter than when I had entered. The Thorsens were not smiling, exactly, but they looked at me expectantly, even hopefully.

I could well imagine that they were feeling raw, exposed, and vulnerable. I had spoken slowly and in small chunks, reading their expressions and not wanting to overwhelm them with information. The brief silences invited them to ask questions. Even though they sat quietly, pondering what had been said, it was important to pause within the flow of our conversation. I had already given them a lot to think about. And I had a lot of ground still to cover.

I took the opportunity to frame the upcoming conversation by watering a seed I had planted.

"A moment ago I said that I want to make sure you receive the best care possible. In addition to all the treatments for this disease, that includes attending to your symptoms and sense of well-being. It also includes offering practical, problem-solving help and emotional support to your family."

I intentionally use the phrase "the best care possible" in my conversations with people early in our relationship as doctor and patient.

When it comes to life-threatening illness, it is the one thing everyone agrees on. If we or someone we love becomes seriously ill, we want the best care possible. So, too, those of us who are doctors want *the best care possible* for our patients. What that phrase means, of course, differs from one person to another. One size does not fit all. Given the Thorsens' palpable apprehension when I entered the room, it felt particularly important to explicitly name my intentions during our first visit.

"I want to find out what the best care possible means for you, in this particular situation, as you and your family look ahead." I looked at each of them in turn, inviting a response. They met my gaze, but neither spoke. They were taking it all in.

I use the expression as a way of starting an open-ended conversation— a nonthreatening way of approaching some scary topics. However, introducing the expression "the best care possible" is not merely a clever expression. It is a way of getting to things that, as a palliative care physician, I really need to know.

Within the panoply of medical specialties, the goal of this new discipline is for patients and families to receive the best care we can collectively deliver. Striving to provide the best care possible provides a

conceptual frame for employing specific palliative treatments and services in the course of a person's illness and care: treating pain, shortness
of breath, or other symptoms; communicating and coordinating services
among different specialties; clarifying goals of care. Each component
would likely contribute to providing the best care for the Thorsens—in
due time.

Today, their focus was on getting through chemotherapy and radiation treatments in preparation for a big operation several months in the
future. We were fully on board in his fight against the disease. And, if the
time were to come, we would be there to help him die gently, as well as
to support Elaine in her caregiving and in her grief.

Whenever circumstances allow, my clinical work begins before I
actually meet a new patient. In addition to reviewing a person's medical history and test results, my habit is to check the administrative part
of their medical chart. I am particularly interested in the demographic
information the individual gave on the hospital's admission forms. As
thin as this information often is, it can help me get a sense of the person's
background and social situation, and it is a way of preparing for a first
encounter.

On the lines following questions of his employment, marital status,
and religion, Mr. Thorsen had written Retired, Married, Catholic. His
responses did not tell me who he is, but it was a start. (They were different from Unemployed, Divorced, No Preference, which my last patient
had written.) The demographics did not provide a clear picture of Mr.
Thorsen but, like the early paint on a canvas or the first day's work of
a sculptor's hammer and chisel, I could begin to glimpse an emerging
shape.

The preparation is useful. In the interview that would follow, I listened closely to what Mr. Thorsen did for a living prior to retiring, how
long he and Elaine had been together before being married (and whether
he had been married before), how active a Catholic he considered himself, and how his religion was affecting his experience of being ill.

When I asked, he said that he had been raised Catholic. "But after what I saw in Vietnam . . . my religion is 'do unto others,' ya know what I mean?" He looked at me and I nodded and told him he was clear.

"I guess you could say we are 'Christmas Catholics.' We go to Mass every Christmas Eve with our children when we are together."

"Easter, too," Elaine added, smiling for the first time.

"Yes"—he chuckled—"on Easter, too," and looked at her affectionately. It struck me that Gerry and Elaine Thorsen were not only husband and wife; they were best friends.

The only way a clinician can become expert in the practice of palliative medicine is one patient at a time.

In meeting a patient in a clinic exam room, or in a hospital room, or across a meeting room conference table, I need not formally examine the person to be attentive to his or her appearance, facial expressions, and body language. Doing so allows me to sense how the person is faring at the moment and enables me to adjust my own pace. I can gauge how much to try to accomplish in a single session and decide how much information and level of detail to convey at this visit. People vary greatly—one from another and from one day to another—in how much they are able to absorb or grapple with in one sitting. If I am to serve them well, I need to read and be responsive to their reactions—their readiness, reluctance, or need for respite.

Of course, it is a process. Clinical care tends to be delivered in discrete episodes: office visits, tests, procedures, hospitalizations. Yet from the perspective of someone who is ill—and their family—care is a process that takes place over time. People's situations evolve as treatments take effect—or not—and as they get better or their condition worsens. Each person's illness has a course. The meaning or interpretation of "the best care possible" may well change over time.

As clinicians, our team must keep clarifying what the best care represents for each patient and family on any given day—and then come as close as we can to delivering it.

Besides the knowledge and skills that come with training and experience, palliative care is a practice that requires commitment. That commitment entails being willing to change course as a person's clinical condition improves or worsens and his or her priorities shift. It includes staying engaged if things go badly. When people are seriously ill, sometimes everyone can do everything right and things can still go miserably wrong.

For many of us, the toughest part of practicing medicine is sometimes feeling powerless to make things a lot better. While it is my professional commitment to give the best care I possibly can, I cannot make things perfect. I wished I could take away the Thorsens' distress and tribulations and suffering that may lie ahead. But this is real life—*their life*. I could, however, commit that our team will accompany them to every extent we can through whatever the future may hold.

By introducing the question of what the best care possible means *for them*, I hoped it might help the Thorsens to retain—or regain—firm personal footing, despite the experience that was enveloping them.

It is easy to lose perspective on the role of medicine relative to personal aspects of life—and important not to let that occur. The moment a person becomes ill, his or her personal priorities tend to be subordinated to medical priorities.

When any of us falls seriously ill, we naturally turn to doctors and hospitals to keep us alive. That is what the health system does best. Applying the advances of medical science and technology, doctors cure deadly infections and keep failing hearts, lungs, livers, or kidneys functioning, or replace failed organs with transplanted ones, or with machines that breathe or beat or filter blood for us.

It is understandable to focus on survival. What is more personal, after all, than staying alive?! But doctors do not have to diminish lifesaving treatments to attend to sensitive, and even intimate, aspects of people's experience. Unfortunately, modern doctors are taught to view sick patients through a lens that primarily sees their medical problems. The problem-based frameworks and clinical assessment procedures that are intended to streamline and focus doctors' attention have become like horses' blinders, keeping the focus straight ahead on diseases and their treatments but constraining a broader view.

From their very first introduction to clinical care, medical students are taught to create a problem list for each patient they see. The problem lists form the table of contents of each patient's medical chart. However, to a person who is living with an incurable illness, life is more than a set of medical problems to be treated. The fundamental nature of illness is not medical; it is personal.

But in health care today, people's personal lives take a backseat to medical treatments. When a person becomes seriously ill, it is likely his or her doctor who will say, "We need to run some important tests and start treatments right away." In that sentence is the tacit message: "Put your personal life on hold."

Of course, for someone with a life-threatening condition, life can't be put on hold for very long. Doctors—including those I train—must be able to use the problem-based approach while also tending to personal realms of people's experience—how the illness affects their self-image, their work, relationships, plans, priorities, hopes, and sense of the future. Doing less in not acceptable.

From the moment of diagnosis, people like Gerry and Elaine Thorsen are at risk of becoming strangers in a strange land. For someone who is seriously ill, today's medical centers can be dizzying technological environments that offer hope and threaten despair. For people whose diseases will not be cured but instead progress despite aggressive treatments, the very places that are meant to provide the best care can become dystopias of discomfort, false promises, and foreboding. By virtue of being treated at Dartmouth-Hitchcock, the Thorsens already had access to the best cancer treatments available. I wanted to help them to retain some perspective on their personal life and priorities.

For the Thorsens, the best care possible would require the right diagnostic tests and treatments for Gerry's pancreatic cancer. The best care would also require meticulous attention to managing his symptoms—pain, breathing difficulties, GI upset, constipation or diarrhea. It would entail someone to coordinate services and appointments; consistent, ongoing, and clear communication; frank discussions of potential problems; and planning about how to prevent crises and what to do if they occur. It would require personal attention and genuine human warmth, an amalgam of technical expertise and tender, loving care.

I began today by establishing some rapport and, hopefully, laying the foundation for a trusting, therapeutic relationship. I was banking capital. There might well come a time when I or another member of our team would draw on that trust in helping the Thorsens balance the potential benefits of further treatments against the risks of making things worse and the known costs to their personal time and quality of life.

Before parting, the Thorsens and I made an appointment to see them in three weeks, the day of their next scheduled oncology clinic visit with Dr. Pipas. I gave them my business card and our Palliative Care Service brochure, pointing out phone numbers and emphasizing that there is always a palliative care physician on call 24/7 if they had an urgent problem.

As I left the Thorsens I was struck by how unique and yet all-too-familiar their experience seemed.

No two people are alike. Even physiologically and medically, no two people with the same diagnoses will have the same manifestations of the disease. Illness is the interaction of a person with a disease. Clinicians I think of as "real doctors" can master the science and problem-solving aspects of medicine and at the same time see each patient as a full, unique person. Unfortunately, these days, authentic doctoring often requires swimming against a powerful current.

In many ways, America's health care system is actually a disease treatment system. The ramifications of this distinction reach far into our society and, inevitably, touch our personal lives. Our nation's medical education system has trained twenty-first-century medical students, residents, and fellows to be diseaseologists. Generalists are scarce, almost quaint. Now we have specialists and subspecialists in medicine and surgery for every categorical malady. There are separate medical and surgical subspecialists in cardiovascular disease and neurovascular disease. Similarly, in addition to general specialists (the phrase has taken on meaning) in oncology and neurology, there are now both medical and surgical subspecialties in neuro-oncology. Indeed subspecialization has occurred in endocrinology, gastroenterology, nephrology, hepatology, dermatology, ophthalmology, psychiatry, and on and on. At the present time, there are disease-specific specialists in basically anything that can go wrong.

In this context, a patient's diagnosis (the "pathology") is the central focus. No single discipline is assigned care of the whole person. Once, when phones still had dials, doctors and their offices were the *de facto* health care delivery system. Through the 1980s and early 1990s primary care physicians still played a central, coordinating role. But times have changed. Today, an internist, family physician, pediatrician, or women's health physician may diagnose a serious condition but is likely to lose regular contact with patients once they step onto the moving walkway leading to treatment.

The discipline of palliative care represents one response of our health care system to the hyper-specialization and fragmentation of care. Our focus in palliative care is on whole persons and their families.

In the twenty-first century health care is delivered by highly specialized teams of professionals, working within complex systems. In the world in which we now live, the best care possible entails more than just having brilliant doctors. It takes a team of people—actually an array of teams—effectively communicating and working together.

Palliative care is an interdisciplinary team approach to care for people with life-threatening conditions, which addresses physical, emotional, social, and spiritual distress and seeks to improve quality of life for the ill person and his or her family. It is important to distinguish the word "interdisciplinary" from "multidisciplinary" in this context. Multidisciplinary care occurs when various professionals from different disciplines assess a patient and write recommendations in the patient's chart. "Interdisciplinary" implies that on a regular basis representatives of those disciplines are in the same room, communicating and collaborating to craft an individualized plan of care. Patients and their families are at the center of the process, whether or not they participate in formal care planning conferences. Their preferences, values, priorities, and styles guide the team's recommendations.

Interdisciplinary teams foster creative collaborations that result in the whole being more than the sum of its parts. Interdisciplinary plans of care tend to be more comprehensive than plans developed through less interactive processes.

Embracing collaborative approaches to care does not diminish the importance of individual clinicians—and especially doctors. In recent years, Medicare and insurance regulations, increasingly complex health care systems, and corporate, for-profit medicine have all diminished the authority of doctors. But even within these complicated systems and subspecialized times—*especially in these systems and times*—doctors have enormous influence on people's care and quality of life. When someone is seriously ill, a good doctor is a mighty thing.

To serve well, doctors need to understand the perspective of the patients and families they serve. What things look and sound like from a clinical perspective can be very different from what they look and sound like—and *feel like*—within the experience of a person and family.

Because, like the Thorsens, every patient and family is unique, to serve people as well as possible, doctors and health systems must make highly individualized and personalized care routine.

And to serve well, doctors must also teach. We must teach patients and families, as well as other clinicians. Indeed, the English word "doctor" comes from the Latin *docere*, to teach. In an academic hospital, clinical practice and clinical teaching are interwoven. Teaching is a privilege and heavy responsibility. In addition to reinforcing the basic science, therapeutic principles, evidence base, and technical skills of medicine, I train young physicians to listen closely, so that they can begin to imagine what patients and families may be feeling as they live through life's most difficult situations.

Part Two

Life-and-Death Decisions

2.

Between Scylla and Charybdis, a Rock and a Hard Place, and the Devil and the Deep Blue Sea

I listened carefully as Mrs. Maxwell's family described their beloved mother, aunt, and grandmother.

We sat in a crowded conference room in the intensive care unit or ICU. Six members of Janice Maxwell's family were present—her daughter, Evie, and her husband, Frank; her son, Ellis, and his wife and their son, Ellis Jr.; and Cici, a niece who lived next door to Mrs. Maxwell. In addition to myself, there was Dr. Carrick Utley, an oncology fellow rotating through our service, Dr. Christine Geffen, Mrs. Maxwell's current attending critical care physician, a consulting neurologist, a nurse practitioner from the cardiology team, the primary nurse taking care of Mrs. Maxwell today, as well as one of the ICU social workers and a chaplain.

Members of two additional specialty teams (infectious disease and cardiothoracic surgery) that had consulted on Mrs. Maxwell's care could not be present. Neither could our patient. Janice Maxwell was being ventilated—breathed for—in ICU room 11. There were important decisions about her care that her family and health care teams needed to discuss this afternoon.

At about two o'clock I had paged Carrick, who was in his second of four weeks with our service, a recently added requirement of Dartmouth's Hematology-Oncology fellowship program. He had spent the morning seeing patients in clinic with Betty Priest, one of our team's nurse practitioners, and Laura Rollano, our social worker. I wanted him to join me for the upcoming ICU family meeting.

We arrived at Mrs. Maxwell's bedside while her family was still gathering in the ICU waiting room. Carrick and I briefly evaluated Mrs. Maxwell. We spoke to her, letting her know who we were and that "we are here to check on you," and touched her hand and her brow. We looked for any response. There was none. We took note of the five IV drips and the current rates of each medication. Carrick jotted data from the monitors, recording her pulse, blood pressure, oxygen saturation, and the settings of her ventilator. He and I discussed her medication dosages and overall condition with her nurse.

At sixty-nine, Mrs. Maxwell's health had not been good for many years. In addition to being overweight, she had high blood pressure for which she took two pills daily, and diabetes for which she took two types of insulin. Each morning she injected a long-acting insulin, and when her finger stick glucose tests were high after meals, she gave herself an injection of short-acting insulin. Until now, however, she had never been seriously ill.

Three weeks ago, Mrs. Maxwell developed a fever and generalized achiness. Then, while sitting at her kitchen table clipping discount coupons from the weekend *Valley News*, she suddenly became blind to anything in her right field of vision and felt dizzy, as if the room were spinning. Her niece, Cici, was upstairs and heard her aunt call out, which Cici described as a loud grunting. When she saw her aunt on the kitchen floor, she immediately called 911 and comforted her until the ambulance arrived and the EMTs (emergency medical technicians) whisked Mrs. Maxwell away to the local emergency department. There the doctor readily diagnosed a stroke, but also astutely recognized the constellation of fever, diffuse aches and pains, and localized neurological deficits as symptoms and signs of endocarditis, a bacterial infection of one or more valves in her heart. The emergency department doctor documented a characteristic rash and small hemorrhages that looked like tiny splinters under Mrs. Maxwell's fingernails. Blood was drawn for laboratory tests, including bacterial cultures, an IV was started, and she was transferred to Dartmouth-Hitchcock Medical Center.

Mrs. Maxwell's infection likely began with a sore on the side of her leg. Now deep in her heart, the blood cultures and echo cardiograms revealed clusters of staphylococcus on the cords and leaflets of her aortic valve that were sending infected debris into her circulation—like microscopic bacterial barnacles swept along in the current. Some landed in her brain where they blocked small arteries and caused sudden symptoms. A few of her symptoms—her dizziness and confusion—initially improved over the first day as spasms in the walls of arteries acutely affected by the emboli gradually relaxed. However, these were not simple blood clots or fragments of atherosclerotic plaques. Each embolus was a minute bit of pus. Everywhere they landed a bacterial infection was sown. Each infected arteriole in the brain's circulation was capable of bleeding. All of this explained Janice Maxwell's sudden loss of vision, the vertigo, and her waxing and waning level of awareness.

Her brain was not the only organ affected by the acute condition. Some of these bacterial emboli landed in the kidneys and various muscles, and some in the tips of the capillaries in her fingertips. But the lesions in her brain were the most dangerous threats to her imminent survival and long-term recovery.

On admission to the hospital Mrs. Maxwell's condition was tenuous. She was sleepy and seemed not to notice her loss of vision to her right. When asked by the nurses and physicians at DHMC, she placidly said she understood where she was. Also, whenever asked, she told them she was not in pain. Within forty-eight hours of her admission to DHMC, Mrs. Maxwell began to improve. Antibiotics seemed to halt the progression of the infections in her heart and brain. As the intravenous medications seeped into tissue fluids throughout her body, the infection and inflammation began to wane everywhere else the bacteria had landed. Her fever subsided. Her condition became less immediately life threatening. She was slightly more alert and able to enjoy a few spoonfuls of applesauce and Jell-O.

At 6:22 the evening of her third hospital day, Mrs. Maxwell suddenly became unresponsive and her breathing became shallow. Her daughter, Evie, and Evie's husband, Frank, had been visiting in her room and, alarmed by the abrupt change, immediately called for Mrs. Maxwell's nurse. The hospital's emergency response team—"HERT team" for short—was called and she was intubated. The critical care fellow stood above Mrs. Maxwell's head as she lay motionless on her back. He opened her mouth with his thumb, slid the blunt metal blade of the laryngoscope over her tongue, lifted her tongue until he could see her larynx in the light of the scope, and passed a plastic tube the width of her index finger through her vocal cords and into her trachea. The other end of that endotrachial tube was then firmly connected to a football-size bag of oxygen, which was then held and rhythmically squeezed by a respiratory therapist who walked alongside Mrs. Maxwell as she was moved, bed and all, to the ICU.

On arrival, an ICU nurse took over "bagging" Mrs. Maxwell, while the respiratory therapist reconnected the endotrachial tube to a mechanical ventilator. Ever since—for the last twenty-two days—the ventilator had generated a breath up to fourteen times a minute, every time four and a half seconds went by without Mrs. Maxwell drawing a breath on her own.

A new CT scan showed a new shower of fifteen or more small strokes. Neurologically, this was a major setback. Although people can improve, sometimes surprisingly, in the early days or even first few weeks after a stroke, the cumulative impact of Mrs. Maxwell's successive strokes portended ill.

From a cardiovascular perspective, she was stable, at least for the moment. But her aortic valve was damaged by the staphylococcal infection and at high risk of failing. And were her aortic valve to fail, the strain on her already stressed heart muscle would likely kill her within minutes. At best, the infection could be suppressed for weeks or even months. Any cure would require surgery to replace her infected aortic valve with a mechanical one (her heart was too large for the bioprosthetic valves made from pig hearts or from human cadavers). Unfortunately, her strokes would preclude the blood thinners that are needed after a mechanical valve replacement to prevent clots and emboli. In this case, anticoagulant medications would almost certainly cause significant bleeding in her brain. It was a damned-if-you-do, damned-if-you-don't situation. Yet, even without those complicating factors, Mrs. Maxwell's other health problems, including diabetes and her five foot, three inch, 280-pound body habitus, led the cardiovascular surgeons to believe she would not survive the surgery. In their written consultation, the CT (cardiothoracic) surgery team did not offer to operate, but suggested continued aggressive medical management and offered to reevaluate in several weeks if her condition improved.

As we met in the ICU conference room on this mid-November afternoon, Mrs. Maxwell's overall medical condition was bleak. Since the day she was urgently transferred to the ICU, she remained minimally conscious. Unlike most patients who require pain and sedative medications to suppress coughing or involuntarily "bucking" the ventilator as it pushes compressed, oxygenated air into their windpipes, she tolerated it all without medication. That was not a hopeful sign.

The large majority of every day she was completely unresponsive, making no movements and lacking any visible response to someone's voice or to being touched. Occasionally, just once or twice during each of the last few days, she made a facial expression or seemed to grip someone's hand, but it was hard for any of the doctors or nurses to tell whether the movements were purposeful or merely due to muscle reflexes.

Dr. Geffen, the critical care specialist currently in charge of her care, consulted our Palliative Care Service. She wanted us to assist Janice Maxwell's family in clarifying goals for her care in the context of her stable but dire condition. On the administrative data collection sheet we use to monitor referrals to our program, "clarify goals of care" is the most commonly indicated reason we are consulted for hospitalized patients. Dr. Geffen hoped we could help the Maxwell family understand and sort through treatment decisions concerning long-term ventilation and medically administered nutrition and hydration that needed to be made.

When I spoke to her, Dr. Geffen described the Maxwells as a devoted family whose members were having difficulty adjusting to the severity of the patient's condition. It was a particularly difficult situation, she felt, because on any given day Mrs. Maxwell was neither improving nor deteriorating. However, the consensus among the medical teams involved in Mrs. Maxwell's care was that her prospects for long-term survival were slim and her prospects for recovering any semblance of independent function slimmer still.

I had briefly met Mrs. Maxwell's daughter, Evie, and son-in-law, Frank, before the afternoon's meeting. About 6:20 the prior evening, I had stopped at her bedside, arriving just as they were leaving. They were both wearing jackets over work clothes. Evie wore a Shaw's supermarket smock and Frank a mustard yellow poplin shirt with his name and the logo of a heating oil company. I introduced myself, briefly explained the role of our palliative care team, and said that I would be involved in the next day's meeting. They acknowledged the gravity of Evie's mother's condition and thanked me for coming by. They apologized for being unable to visit longer, explaining that they needed to get home to their teenage son and household. Brief as it was, the encounter set a friendly tone for the conversations to come.

This afternoon, Carrick and I stood with the Maxwell family for a few minutes in the busy inner corridor of the unit. As an earlier meeting was ending and people filed out of the ICU's only conference room, I exchanged polite smiles and nods with several nurses, residents, and a housekeeper who passed by. Our palliative care team members are familiar faces and names in the ICU, a result of working closely with the critical care teams.

Connie Pollock, the ICU social worker, had text-paged each of the doctors and the nurse practitioner involved a few minutes earlier, reminding us of the meeting. Now, she and I acted as ushers to get everyone into the room. Members of Mrs. Maxwell's family took seats around one end of the long, old, blond oak conference table, sitting in sturdy, stackable gray plastic chairs that are ubiquitous throughout the medical center. The walls were a cluttered mosaic of flyers announcing upcoming conferences and a going-away party for a nurse, and quality-improvement project posters with graphed monthly scores of ventilator acquired pneumonias and intravenous line infections from August to October. On a large whiteboard that occupied half of one wall, hand-written diagrams and formulas for calculating vascular resistance gave evidence of a recent teaching session.

As soon as everyone was settled, Connie nodded to me and I spoke.

"Hello, everybody. For those of you I haven't yet met, I'm Dr. Byock, I am with the Palliative Care Service. Since there are a number of us here, I suggest we start by introducing ourselves to one another." I turned to the woman on my right who nodded in recognition.

"Thanks, Dr. Byock. I am Evie Chandler, Maxie's daughter."

"I am Frank Chandler, Evie's husband, and Maxie's favorite son-in-law." He smiled beneath his Red Sox hat. His comment generated muted chuckles from other members of the family. One muttered it was only because Frank was her only son-in-law.

The light but respectful tone persisted as each person, in turn, family and clinicians alike, gave his or her name and relationship to

Mrs. Maxwell and her care. Thus, the meeting began. Each member of Mrs. Maxwell's family, doctors, and staff introduced themselves in turn. Then it was time for me to get to the purpose of our gathering.

There were two decisions that needed to be made—if not today, then very soon. One concerned whether or not to place a tracheostomy tube for long-term mechanical ventilation. The other was whether to place a PEG (percutaneous endoscopic gastronomy) tube for nutrition and hydration. Both procedures required formal consent. Assuring a clinically sound and ethical process for making decisions about Mrs. Maxwell's care was the immediate reason for meeting. Of course, it was not just the risks and potential benefits of these procedures that warranted discussion, but also her overall condition, prognosis, and care in general that needed to be discussed. As the facilitator of the meeting, I felt it was important for the discussion to be grounded in the life and person of Mrs. Maxwell.

The clinical teams knew an enormous amount about her organ functions and the intimate anatomy of her brain and heart, but none of us had ever met her before her stroke. We had spoken *to* her, but never *with* her.

"We have a number of things to discuss today about Mrs. Maxwell's condition and at least two treatments to consider. But since I have not previously met you and have never had the opportunity to meet before her illness, I thought it would be helpful to get a sense of who she is. I know that she is widowed and owns a bakery. But that is all. I do not even know where she grew up. So, if you don't mind, I wonder if we could spend just a few minutes talking about her as a person: her history, what she has done in the remote and recent past, and the things she likes and dislikes."

Evie began. She described Mrs. Maxwell—whom everyone affectionately called "Maxie"—as a dynamo. Anticipating our unspoken prejudices, she remarked that people were surprised that someone as big as her mother could have so much energy and be in constant motion.

She had grown up in Albany, New York, and moved with her family to Vermont when she was in high school. She and her future husband, Elbert, met in their early twenties, when both were working at a summer camp in the Green Mountains. After he returned from World War II, he went to work as a machinist. She baked for several area restaurants, but was primarily mother to the couple's son and daughter. Elbert died suddenly in 1989. With their children grown and on their own, Janice started her own catering business a year after Elbert's death. She also found the time to chair the board of the county's food bank and organize its holiday collection drives.

In decades past, the town's police chief and school officials knew that Janice and Elbert Maxwell were always willing to take in a troubled child or teenager for a few days—and sometimes longer—until other arrangements could be made. A few of those kids stayed a lot longer and became members of the extended Maxwell family.

Every member of that family present at the meeting described Janice Maxwell as the best mother, aunt, sister, and grandmother anyone could have. She was constantly calling and asking about things they were doing. It was not because she was nosy—she was genuinely interested and very much a part of all of their lives. Her granddaughter and niece said that Maxie knew everything about them: what classes they were taking, when their exams or major papers were due, what they were doing in sports and clubs, even what boys they were dating! Cici said that she had taught Maxie to text and they exchanged at least two or three messages a day.

I thanked them for their descriptions. It had taken all of six minutes, but in that brief time those of us who knew Mrs. Maxwell only as a patient got to see her as a whole and vibrant person. I think we all better understood her family's predicament: their hope for her to live, their burden of decisions, their pressing fear and looming grief. The few minutes of conversation would enable us to better care for her and support all of them.

I asked the critical care doctors to review Mrs. Maxwell's current condition and the rationale for both procedures. Dr. Geffen described her condition as generally stable, but was careful to add, "She continues to be critically ill." She explained that a tracheostomy involves surgically placing a short plastic tube through the skin of a patient's neck and into her trachea, just below her larynx (or Adam's apple). The "trach" would protect Mrs. Maxwell's vocal cords and the narrow portion of her windpipe. The PEG involves surgically placing a plastic tube about the width of a fountain pen through a patient's abdominal wall to deliver nutrition and hydration directly into her stomach. The consulting neurologists explained that if the infection could be halted, it could take many weeks to see improvement in Mrs. Maxwell's level of awareness and function, but that she would likely require substantial care for the rest of her life.

No one was suggesting that any of her current treatments be withdrawn—at least not yet. But there was an unspoken awareness that, at some point, more treatment might not be what was best for her. At some point, we would likely need to discuss how she could die. Probably not today, but in all likelihood soon.

Even without stating that a patient is dying, by broaching the possibility—suggesting that it would be reasonable to not escalate treatments further if the condition were to worsen or even consider withdrawing life-sustaining treatments—twenty-first-century doctors are in a difficult situation. People come to doctors to save their lives, not to be helped to die. In these times, doctors may risk being fired by a family for suggesting it would be reasonable to let a person die. People demand second, third, fourth, and fifth opinions. For the persistent, there is always a more famous medical center where they have "real specialists" for this or that condition.

It is not just me and my ilk of palliative care physicians who are at risk of being fired. I have seen highly respected surgeons, intensivists, and oncologists fired from cases by angry patients or families for suggesting that further treatment would be futile. Often care is simply transferred to a doctor willing to persist. If that is not possible, a medical center's ethics committee gets involved in an effort to reach agreement. Only if this course of action fails to resolve the conflict is the matter brought to a court for a judge to hear. This process can take months. Not uncommonly, the patient dies before any decisions are made.

Savvy and assertive advocacy is a powerful and often essential factor in getting the best care possible. To be effective, advocacy must be rooted in the reality of what is possible and directed at obtainable goals; otherwise, it can be counterproductive.

It is important to make sure doctors don't give up treatments too soon on someone. Without ill intention or incompetence on the part of doctors, occasionally people with complex but treatable conditions are told that there is nothing else to be done to extend their lives when, in fact, there may be. It is worthwhile to be wary of a single physician's sophistication, experience, or personal values—or a single medical center's technical capacity—and not let either unduly limit a patient's treatment options.

At the same time, it is important to acknowledge the biological limits of treatment. Even the most savvy and assertive individuals who are incurably ill—including those who choose all aggressive treatments—eventually die.

In my experience, when a patient's disease is clearly progressing and complications are accumulating, the condition itself serves as a counselor for both the ill person and his or her family. By continually eroding quality of life or requiring ever more medications to lessen suffering, a person's deteriorating state of health eventually brings even the most reluctant of their friends and relatives to realize that the person they love is dying.

I've learned it is better to earn people's trust and stay involved. Our team earns trust, first, by attending to patients' most urgent needs, such as managing pain or other distress. Second, concomitantly, we build relationships by regularly offering information about the patient's condition, explaining what it means, and responding to questions in whatever depth patients and families desire. As changes warrant, "explaining what it means" encompasses discussion of the implications of the patient's current condition on the person's survival and the prospects for rehabilitation and likely long-term ability to function, along with corresponding caregiving needs. "Explaining what it means" is typically both labor- and time-intensive. That's okay. Communication is not ancillary or a chore in palliative care; rather, it is the core therapeutic medium of our discipline. The time it takes palliative clinicians to effectively listen, convey information, and respond to questions and concerns is not time taken from our medical practice; it *is* the practice.

This palliative approach of building trust by managing symptoms, attending to family concerns, therapeutic communication, and continuity is intensive care of a different sort. It is certainly expensive, in terms of clinicians' time and energy, but it is also better in the long run by being both effective and efficient. In this manner palliative care complements critical care by enhancing quality (and patient and family satisfaction). Expensive as this approach to care is, compared with being at odds with patients and families, and having to resolve and manage conflict, best practices of this sort usually consume a lot less time and resources.

Intensive, lifesaving treatments were essential to the best possible care when Mrs. Maxwell had arrived at the local emergency department, was transferred to DHMC's emergency department, was admitted to the hospital, and was later transferred to the ICU. However, on the day we met, things were different—or, in this instance, not different enough. Her prognosis was increasingly bleak. Her family was struggling to determine what the best care for Mrs. Maxwell was *now*. We all were. They still hoped for a cure. Yet within the last week or so, most members of her family had come to realize that it wasn't going to happen. Still, it is one thing to know that someone you love is dying and another thing to say it.

These were literally life-and-death decisions. Without the ventilator to breathe for her, she would likely die within a few minutes. Without medically administered nutrition, she would die within weeks. Without medically administered fluid, she would die within days. A decision regarding the tracheostomy was most pressing. Eventually the inflated plastic cuff around the endotrachial tube would cause pressure sores and scarring around the lining of her windpipe. As a general guideline, it is prudent to perform "a trach" after two weeks of intubation, and at twenty-two days, a decision was needed: to proceed or to withdraw the tube and, therefore, disconnect her from the ventilator.

I thought to myself that it would have been helpful for her family if Mrs. Maxwell had an advance directive on file. Advance directives— a living will or a durable power of attorney for health care—are legal documents in which people can state their preferences for care if they are seriously ill and not able to make decisions for themselves. If one existed, I could have used it to inform the conversation of the meeting. As it was, in common with nearly 75 percent of adults in America, she had never completed one.

Mrs. Maxwell's condition and the treatments being considered exemplified the situation these documents were created to address.

A durable power of attorney for health care document formally names a person to speak for you if you are seriously ill and unable to speak for yourself. A living will provides information about your preference for treatments if you become terminally ill and are unable to make your own decisions.

Over time, these documents increasingly have been combined as two sections of single forms. Advance directives are legally recognized in every state. And states generally recognize documents completed in another state.

In New Hampshire, where Mrs. Maxwell was being cared for, by state law a power of attorney document is necessary to confer formal decision-making authority for an incapacitated adult to a spouse, child, or parent. Without such a document, no individual had final authority to make important decisions about Mrs. Maxwell's treatments. Nevertheless, as physicians responsible for her care, we turned to Mrs. Maxwell's family to help us clarify goals of care and, as partners in the process, of making these critical decisions. In fact, even when an advance directive exists, and while recognizing the authority of the individuals appointed in the document, we try to foster agreement among participating family members in defining each patient's goals of care.

I decided to see if Mrs. Maxwell's family had a sense of what she would have written in an advance directive. I asked what family members thought Mrs. Maxwell would say about her care, if she could speak for herself today.

Evie looked down at the table and chuckled to herself. Then she raised her head and spoke, recalling an occasion when her mother had talked about a neighbor who had suffered a paralyzing stroke. "I remember Mom said that she wouldn't want to live if she couldn't cook, eat, and 'wipe my own ass!'" Hearty laughter signaled broad agreement.

Ellis, Evie's brother, said that he was sure their mother would think that lying in an ICU this long was ridiculous and would want to be put out of her misery. Frank and Ellis's wife both nodded. Ellis Jr., who I guessed to be in his mid-twenties and had explained during the introductions that he had lived with Maxie during his senior year in high school, agreed that she would not want to be kept alive on machines.

For a few minutes, there was a gathering consensus that Mrs. Maxwell would prefer to die gently and I thought that perhaps today was the day. But then her niece, Cici, who had been quiet since the discussion of Mrs. Maxwell's history, spoke up.

"It isn't right just to let her die," she said softly, looking down at her hands held together resting on the conference table. "Only God can take a life."

The comment blew through the room like a winter wind through an open door. Around the table, the atmosphere suddenly chilled and people gathered their shoulders to their necks and looked down.

I later learned that Cici had battled alcoholism and drugs during her own teenage years. A little over two years ago she joined AA and had been clean and sober since. She had embraced Christianity as part of her 12-step program. Maxie had been a big part of Cici's recovery.

Evie broke the uncomfortable stillness. "Cici, no one is talking about killing Maxie. But she is not getting well."

"But she still can. They haven't said she absolutely can't get better. Other people in her condition have gotten better—even after years in a coma. Miracles happen, you know."

Miracles do happen. Sometimes against all odds and without explanation deathly ill people suddenly become better. There's no denying it—and I wouldn't want to. It seems the nature of miracles that they happen rarely. Still, who is to say a miracle could not happen here?

If I had known the Maxwell family better—if I had had the time to earn their trust—I might have taken a more assertive tact. I might have asked Cici to consider that Mrs. Maxwell could have died abruptly that morning in their kitchen and that her initial survival was already a miracle. I might have suggested that the past few weeks have given her and her family precious time to spend with her aunt and the chance to support one another. If I had known Cici better and had been more aware of her devoutly Christian beliefs, I might have asked her to share with me her understanding of how people whom God loves eventually die. I might have gently confirmed that she believed that God loved her aunt Maxie. When she said, "Yes, of course God loves her," I would have asked Cici if it were possible that God's will was already being done?

But on this day, having just met them all, saying any of these things risked going too far. The question of miracles effectively foreclosed any consideration of allowing her to die today.

The tenderness of Cici's plea and her family's need to support her in her devotion to Maxie were apparent. I tried to assure Cici that no one was trying to play God or in any way lessen her aunt's chances of getting well. I said we were all trying to respect her wishes, recognizing that even with intensive care Maxie was at very high risk of dying. Cici made eye contact with me briefly, but mostly looked at her hands resting on the conference table. She did not seem angry, just sad and hurting.

As the meeting drew to a close, the family and we assembled professionals came to the decision to give treatments a little more time and jointly agreed to proceed with the tracheostomy and PEG tube. Both would be done in the operating room the next day.

With those major decisions made, I asked if there were any limitations on her treatments that the family would want to set. I specifically discussed CPR and the use of vasopressors, medications that tightened arteries and made the heart beat faster and stronger, but at the cost of straining the heart and other organs. Her family—with Evie and Ellis taking the lead—decided that treatments should not escalate any further. This meant that if her blood pressure dropped due to a new infection or sudden heart problem, she would not be treated with "pressors." If her heart suddenly stopped, no one would push on her chest and no electrical shocks would be administered to her heart. Cici sat in quiet acquiescence during that part of the discussion. She seemed satisfied that she had prevailed in a room of her elders and was protecting her aunt from a premature death.

I assured members of her family that our team would be checking on Mrs. Maxwell daily and doing whatever we could to enhance her comfort. I was scheduled to be the physician on service this Thanksgiving, so I said I would be looking in on her personally. I asked if they would like us to bring a CD player and her favorite music to her room. Yes, they said that would be good. "She loves Elvis Presley and Johnny Cash," Ellis said. "And anything by Garth Brooks," Cici added.

"Okay," I said, "I know we have some Elvis and Johnny Cash. I will have one of our volunteers bring a boom box to her room and a selection of music. Feel free to bring more. Please also bring a few photos of Maxie if you have them. I would love to see a picture of her in happier times. Pictures will help all of us to know her a bit better."

We agreed and arranged to meet again at three p.m. on the Tuesday afternoon after Thanksgiving. I thanked them all for coming and we slowly dispersed.

I agreed with the decision we reached as a group, but I was not entirely at peace with what had occurred. I wondered what the meeting looked like from Carrick's perspective.

He and I would discuss the content and process of the meeting later in the day and I reflected on the things I wanted him to learn from what had transpired. The meeting had included key elements of physician-family communication and shared decision-making. Well and good. Yet the Tuesday after Thanksgiving was twelve days from now; it seemed a very long time in the future. I knew, after all, that Mrs. Maxwell was not going to survive. It would be a fair criticism to say that in concluding the meeting as we did—*as I did*—we had kicked the can down the road. It would be easy to argue that the operations she was about to undergo were pointless. Carrick and I would discuss the collective, resource implications of this situation, the other patients who might benefit from that ICU bed—since as usual, the ICU was full—and the thousands of people across the country in similar predicaments. There are 3,228 hospitals with ICUs and a total of over 67,000 ICU beds in our country, and many are occupied by people who have been critically ill for weeks on end.

I planned to explain to Carrick my assessment that being more directive today would have been heavy-handed. To some of the family, if only out of loyalty to Cici, it might have felt rushed. To Cici, it might have felt cruel. Of course, as a physician in such situations, I never know where the breaking point lies, where trust will fracture, giving way to conflict, unless I take a step too far.

In fact, despite the pressure on health care resources, we could continue to treat Mrs. Maxwell for her kidney failure, respiratory failure, and heart failure, even if it were only to give her family time to adjust to the reality that she could not get well. In our hospital, on this day, as in hospitals across the country, there were sufficient resources to do so. The financing of American health care well supports such treatments. In many parts of the world ICU beds and ventilators are in scarce supply. Had Mrs. Maxwell been intubated at all in those countries, it would be necessary now to remove life support and allow her to die. But not in our hospital, not in the United States, not today. Not yet.

This clinical scenario is familiar to anyone who practices in hospitals and ICUs, particularly within referral centers. Of course, Mrs. Maxwell's situation is unique. She is a one-of-a-kind person with a unique life story. Still, the basic set of circumstances that had befallen Mrs. Maxwell and her family occurs multiple times a month in our medical center's ICUs and multiple times every day in hospitals across the United States.

As my mind's eye scanned the two main ICUs at Dartmouth-Hitchcock, I saw snapshots of several other patients and families who were currently in similar predicaments:

————

WANDA SMITH is twenty-seven years old. A week ago she had an operation to remove a large tumor that had wrapped around her uterus, bladder, and rectum. There is now no sign of cancer, meaning she is likely cured. It would be a remarkable success, except that after the twelve-hour surgery, she has yet to wake up and is still not breathing on her own.

DONALD GILBERT is a seventy-five-year-old husband, father, and grandfather who suffered a stroke while shaving one morning. A clot formed in his atherosclerotic middle cerebral artery, one of the main branches of the carotid artery, and caused mechanical blockage and spasm of the arteries beyond the clot. Thrombolytic medications administered by the stroke team in the emergency department failed to improve his condition. He cannot speak and makes few intelligible responses. Mr. Gilbert has been able to come off the ventilator twice. Both times he breathed on his own for fewer than twenty-four hours before a sudden deterioration—likely a mucus plug in a bronchus or aspiration of saliva—resulted in the HERT team being called and the endotrachial tube being urgently reinserted. Now, as his older brother has observed at his bedside, "he looks tuckered out."

IDA SAMUELS is sixty-two and has battled lung cancer for the past three and a half years. Our team knows her well and has followed her in the clinic and during hospitalizations in conjunction with the thoracic oncology team. Mrs. Samuels has never wanted to discuss her wishes for care if she were to die because she felt doing so would violate her commitment to being positive. For the same reason, she has never filled out advance directives. She was a highly motivated patient. As soon as cancer was diagnosed, she quit smoking. She went through aggressive chemotherapy and respiratory therapy, and had half of her left lung removed. Within a year, the cancer returned in her lung, lymph nodes, and bones. That was when she was referred to us, nearly eighteen months ago. She had already lived much longer than most people with similar conditions. Since then she has spent weeks in the hospital from pneumonia that kept recurring due to narrowing of the bronchus—or windpipe—to her remaining left lung. Seven weeks ago, using a fiber-optic bronchoscope, a pulmonologist placed a stent, which widened the opening. Now, however, pneumonia was back with a vengeance and she was back in the ICU. In addition to the pneumonia, there is infected fluid around her lung—a condition called empyema—which required a chest tube to be placed through her skin, between her left lower ribs, to continually drain the space between her lung and chest wall. She is on a ventilator, sedated, and paralyzed because she was obviously suffering and thrashing against the ventilator. She has an associated bacterial bloodstream infection that is keeping her blood pressure low and requiring low doses of vasopressor medications.

———

KEVIN HARDY is a forty-two-year-old man who had a sudden cardiac arrest at the gym. Bystanders performed CPR and the EMTs were able to reestablish a pulse. Once at DHMC he underwent emergency cardiac catheterization. A cardiologist was able to locate the blockage and open the clogged artery with a small balloon and place a small expansile stent that looks like a Chinese finger trap. The angioplasty was successful. His heart problem was solved. To minimize swelling and damage to his brain, his body was cooled to 33° centigrade (91.4° Fahrenheit). Two days later, after slowly rewarming him to 37° centigrade (98.6° Fahrenheit), he remains densely comatose with no sign of neurological recovery.

———

AND THEN THERE IS MRS. WALLACE in one of the slightly larger, corner rooms. Her story and her husband's devotion had already made an indelible mark on me and on many of us taking care of her. At age seventy-eight Mrs. Wallace had made good use of twentieth-century medicine. She survived breast cancer in 1989 and went on to have bilateral hip replacements and coronary artery bypass surgery. She played golf and snowshoed every year and felt well until early last spring—it might have been in mid-April, as she told the intern who took her history on admission to the hospital. She had felt tired for days on end and lost her appetite. Blood tests her doctor ordered showed an alarmingly high white blood cell count and a bone marrow biopsy confirmed that she had a treatable lymphoma.

During the rest of the spring and early summer Mrs. Wallace successfully completed three rounds of chemotherapy, tolerating recurring episodes of mouth sores and loss of hair. By midsummer she felt like her old self. However, in August she began slurring her speech and dozing off in the middle of the day, even at meals. Her thyroid was normal. Scans of her brain showed some nonspecific white matter changes. A lumbar puncture—also called a spinal tap—confirmed that there was lymphoma in her cerebral spinal fluid and brain. It was no longer curable.

By then Mrs. Wallace was able only to open her eyes briefly when her name was called. She occasionally clasps a hand placed in hers. Her husband of fifty-seven years, retired Army Colonel William Wallace, lovingly cares for her at their home with the help of privately hired nurses' aides. He calls the ambulance whenever she runs a fever and, as a result, she has been hospitalized four times throughout the late summer and fall.

Mrs. Wallace had a PEG tube placed nearly three weeks ago. She has been in the hospital ever since. The procedure of placing the PEG tube went smoothly. However, Mrs. Wallace's body would not tolerate even a fraction of the amount of nutrient solution (similar to baby formula) required to meet the normal caloric needs of a person of her height and weight. Her intestinal tract seemed inert, unable to move or absorb the liquid being dripped into her stomach. Whenever the rate of formula was increased, she developed diarrhea. She also ran "high residuals," meaning that fluid was just pooling in her stomach and not moving through. Additionally, and more problematically, despite being kept propped at 30 degrees or higher, Mrs. Wallace developed recurrent episodes of coughing that were clearly the result of formula refluxing up her esophagus and down her windpipe. Now she is back in the ICU with florid aspiration pneumonia, once again intubated and on a ventilator. Mr. Wallace is a constant presence at her side.

Each of these cases is unique—one-of-a-kind individuals and circumstances. Yet there are discernible themes.

To remain alive, each of these people will need protection of their airway, and very likely prolonged ventilation, as well as medically administered nutrition and hydration. In each case the chance of recovering function is remote. It is not just that the prospects are slim that the ill person will work, drive, or even walk again. The chances are infinitesimally small that any of these people will ever again perform the most basic elements of self-care: eliminating, washing, brushing one's own teeth, combing one's own hair, and feeding oneself.

Their dependency does not diminish their worthiness of our caring, but it is relevant to the medical treatment decisions that need to be made. Dependency alone is not a reason to withdraw life-prolonging treatment. Quadriplegic people are dependent on others for the most basic elements of care, but most achieve a satisfying "new normal" and many lead active, productive lives. In contrast, none of the ICU patients I just described will ever again enjoy a meal or a conversation, read a book, watch a movie, surf the Web, or take a drive. The distinction is valid. People may disagree about what quality of life is worth sustaining and there is far from a social consensus. But for each individual, it is relevant to consider what quality of life the person, *himself or herself*, would consider worth sustaining. I contend that the combination of a life-threatening illness, complete physical dependence, and a quality of life that is devoid of value *to the person whose life it is* constitutes reasonable rationale for decision-makers to allow a person to die.

Of course, to families in pain things like ethical analyses and rationale, clinical categories and prognostic indicators all seem irrational and irrelevant.

Before his stroke, Mr. Gilbert's family was looking forward to spending Christmas together in Hilton Head, a dual celebration of the holiday and their fiftieth wedding anniversary. Mr. Hardy, the forty-two-year-old man "saved" by CPR, is the principal of a middle school in New Hampshire's Lakes Region. After his cardiac arrest, the entire town organized vigils and meetings and draped trees and telephone poles with white ribbons in his honor. Wanda Smith, who has yet to wake up from her cancer surgery, is the mother of a twenty-two-month-old son. Her husband and parents and brothers and sisters are bereft, cannot envision a future without her, and rarely leave her side.

Mrs. Samuels's son and his wife and young daughter visit every weekend, though they only stay for a short time. They live in Connecticut and have been kept at a distance both literally and figuratively by his domineering mother. Now that her lung cancer has progressed and she is insensate in the ICU, they feel conflicted. They agree that she would never want to give up, but they cannot bear to see her suffer and feel that in her current physical state, she is already dead. Colonel and Mrs. Wallace have six children, eight grandchildren, and two great-grandchildren, at least four of whom are in the ICU waiting room at all times. The colonel is always at her side, stroking her arms and legs with lotion and talking to her softly. Every day, with an almost childlike innocence that is in contrast to his engineering accomplishments, he asks the nurses and doctors about new treatments for lymphoma that friends have suggested or he has read about.

Often I think that if a family could hear the voice of the person who is critically ill, it would help them come to a sound decision. But even that would not be a panacea. Making these decisions is sometimes just as hard when people can speak for themselves.

Carrick and I stride past the corner room of Ralph Barker, a chronically critically ill patient in the ICU who is also in a difficult situation, except that Ralph makes his own decisions. I met Ralph (he doesn't like to be called Mr. Barker) over two months earlier, when the Palliative Care Service was asked by the Critical Care Service to help Ralph and his family clarify goals for his care.

Ralph is fifty-six years old, just a few years younger than I am, but a role of the genetic dice left him diabetic, prone to autoimmune diseases, and chronically ill. His kidneys stopped working when he was forty-nine and his lungs are scarred from inflammation and repeated infections. He has chronic colitis with diarrhea and ulcerating skin sores. He needs daily dressing changes to ulcers on his legs and back, daily colostomy care, and kidney dialysis three times a week. He's mostly confined to bed or a special wheelchair, because he lost his right leg to a bone infection a few years and more than two hundred pounds ago. Despite all this, he had been enjoying his life at home, mostly thanks to his devoted, selfless, and utterly exhausted wife, Sallie.

One day in early September, Ralph suddenly became septic; a profound infection dropped his blood pressure and ability to breathe. He almost died in the ambulance, but after two weeks of antibiotics, mechanical ventilation, and round-the-clock nursing care, Ralph is once again stable. Sort of. Now he has a tracheostomy and still needs a ventilator at night to breathe. Ralph isn't dying today, but he is dying.

He is also suffering. Above all, Ralph says he doesn't want to die. He's never wanted to think about dying and hates when we bring up the subject. He's never completed an advance directive giving anyone formal authority to speak for him if—but really it is *when*—he becomes unable to speak for himself.

Every time I see him, he pleads for two things: for me to prescribe a medicine to make him feel better and for me to send him home.

Panicked anxiety makes him feel breathless even when his oxygen levels are fine. Unless he's somnolent, he craves more doses of sedative medication, but that just makes his breathing worse and makes the prospect of going home an ever-more-distant mirage.

He's never told Sallie or any of his doctors how he would want to be taken care of if he couldn't get well. It is no wonder she feels overwhelmed. As if death were optional, Ralph wants everything possible done to prolong his life, including CPR when his heart eventually stops. He repeatedly tells us he wants to live and go home. Instead, he's confined to the ICU by failing organ systems and the choice he's made to accept technological support to stay alive. In reality, state-of-the-art treatments can't restore anything resembling physical health for Ralph. Since he isn't interested in exploring emotional or spiritual ways through his thorny predicament, all any of us seems able to do is prolong his dying.

In her book *Refuge*, Terry Tempest Williams tells the story of her mother's life with illness. One day, during the last months of her life, Williams's mother reflected, "Dying doesn't cause suffering. Resistance to dying does." I think of this insight often as I meet with and listen closely to people like Ralph, as well as families of people who are critically ill.

People with a sick relative or close friend sometimes ask me how someone would know if they and their family are in this sort of predicament in which resistance to dying is causing suffering. While I am loathe to give advice that can be misapplied to a particular person or specific condition, there are some conservative generalizations I can offer.

If your husband's cancer has continued to grow after the first surgery and radiation, and two or three successive chemotherapy regimens, you may be getting close. The hard truth is that oncologists use their best drugs first. The answers to other questions can help estimate how close: Has the cancer spread to multiple places, including one or more of his bones, liver, lungs, or brain? Has he developed blood clots, despite being on anticoagulants? Has he lost weight? How many weeks has it been since he had an appetite? How much help has he been needing to get around, climb stairs, even bathe?

If your mother has been in the ICU for two or more weeks and things are not getting progressively better, you may be in this predicament. Long ICU stays tend to be worrisome from a prognostic standpoint. Is she requiring a ventilator, or CVVH (continuous kidney dialysis) or vasopressor medications? When a patient has been in the ICU for a long time, each of these treatments is a telling indication of persistent organ failure. Count the number of "lines"—IV, arterial catheters, internal monitors—the number of tubes training internal cavities, the number of wound dressings, the number of antibiotics, the number of sedatives she requires. The higher the numbers, the more seriously ill people are.

To be clear: I am generalizing and there are exceptions to everything I have just described. However, if these situations sound familiar, you and your family may already be faced with balancing the quest to live against the quantity of suffering that accompanies resistance to dying.

People who are physically healthy avoid talking about dying, partly by assuming it will be easier to discuss such matters "when the time comes." Yet, people who are sick and their families discover that it doesn't always get easier. As illness progresses, it sometimes gets harder. Sometimes even bringing the subject up can feel disloyal, a betrayal of a pact to get better.

These are as serious and unfunny as any situations I know. Yet the most apt description I know for this predicament comes from the late comedienne Gilda Radner. Her 1970s *Saturday Night Live* persona, Rose-anne Roseannadanna, famously observed about life in general, "If it's not one thing, it's another thing. But it's always something." Years later, she was diagnosed with ovarian cancer, underwent extensive treatments and experienced a sustained remission, and became an outspoken, effective advocate for people living with cancer. She chose *It's Always Something* for the title of her book about living with cancer. Gilda Radner died of the disease in 1989.

Everyone dies of something. Every time a new complication develops, the doctors will assign it a name, giving you another diagnosis. It may be a new infection, or a new source of bleeding, or clotting (and sometimes both at once). Each diagnosis has a potential treatment, which the doctors will dutifully tell you about—if you haven't already looked it up online.

Yet when someone's underlying illness is progressing or their general condition leaves them weak and with little chance of turning things around, every decision to treat a potentially lethal problem means the person will have to eventually succumb to something else. The question then becomes: What would be an acceptable way for you—or the person you love so much—to die?

That's the question all of us are eventually called to wrestle with for ourselves and for the people we love most in life. As a palliative care physician, it is my job to help people in these unenviable situations to clarify options and make whatever decisions are best for them.

Carrick and I walked from the ICU through automatic double doors onto an inner, staff-only corridor. Except for a housekeeper at the far end of the hall, we were alone. For a while we walked without speaking, each of us still pondering the meeting and wondering what we would say to the other. About a hundred yards from our office, I said, "This job will keep you humble."

Carrick laughs respectfully and after a few steps farther, adds, "But then, as I have heard you say, 'We are just here to serve.'"

"Aha! You have been paying attention." I laughed with him. Humor and camaraderie are good tonics for irony. As a physician, sometimes being "here to serve" means offering the best of one's mind and heart without being attached to what happens, at least not overly attached.

"You know the other thing I often say? 'It is not about us,'" I say. It is a remark without irony, one best made in private—senior physician confiding to a senior physician-in-training. I spoke in the tradition of a profession that has through the centuries passed the craft and art of practice from one generation to the next.

As a doctor teaching other doctors, I deliberately call attention to the pitfall of developing an inflated sense of our own importance. Doctors are important. But ultimately, it is not about us. After all, the sole rationale for our profession is the well-being of others, primarily the patients we serve. At the same time, I try to instill—and model—the value and capacity of being gentle with oneself. Ultimately, no human being can fully control what happens to another. Some things are beyond the grasp of medicine. We can, however, be of service. We can show up, bringing whatever benefits science and technology have to offer, while never losing focus on the persons we serve. That has to be enough.

Sitting around the conference table in the Palliative Care office nibbling on grapes and cookies left over from a No One Alone volunteer meeting, Carrick and I debriefed each other about the dynamics of the meeting. I explain why I said what I did—and why I didn't say more. It had been a hard conversation for Mrs. Maxwell's family to have. Carrick also had the sense that if we had applied directed pressure, we would likely have pushed Cici beyond an emotional breaking point and possibly evoked anger in others. Tincture of time was called for.

Family members I have spoken with months after such meetings have said that during the discussion of treatment decisions—with the very life of their wife or husband, mother or father, sister or brother, son or daughter hanging in the balance—they felt their head spinning, their heart breaking, and their world coming apart. Some have told me that they could not hear what was being said. Some could hear the information but only understand it intellectually, or the words were clear but it felt unreal. One man described feeling unsteady, as if walking in a canoe, unable to take a step or make a decision one way or the other.

That Tuesday after Thanksgiving never came for Mrs. Maxwell. Instead, her family and doctors reconvened at one p.m. on Sunday of the holiday weekend. At about 3:45 Friday morning she stopped triggering the ventilator at all, and her legs and arms stiffened and rotated into a "decerebrate posture," well recognized by doctors and nurses as an ominous sign. It signaled that pressure was rapidly building inside her head causing downward force on her brain and pushing her brain stem against the bony ridge of the circular opening at the base of her skull, which, in turn, causes normally autonomic functions like breathing to stop. The process is called herniation, and it is lethal.

The neurosurgery resident on call was urgently paged to consult and administered IV mannitol, a medication that draws fluid out of the brain, dehydrating it to decrease swelling. An emergency CT scan showed new bleeding and swelling in the right side of her brain, which shifted the rest of her brain downward and to the left. The neurosurgeons then emergently took Mrs. Maxwell to the operating room and installed a drain through her scalp and skull and into the pocket of blood in the right parietal lobe of her brain to stem the buildup of pressure. This halted the impending herniation of her brain and her imminent death.

Evie had been called at 5:20 Friday morning with news of her mother's turn for the worse and, in spite of the group's decision not to escalate treatments further, gave permission for the scans and subsequent surgery. I saw Evie later in the morning, when her mother had just returned to the ICU from the operating room, and again on Saturday afternoon after completing the rest of my rounds. She had taken a leave from her job managing the deli of a large supermarket and was spending most of the time at the hospital. Ellis and his wife and son were visiting as well. Dr. Geffen was no longer the critical care attending physician for Mrs. Maxwell, but I spoke with Dr. Rashid, the critical care fellow, who knew Mrs. Maxwell's case and her family well, and we arranged with the family to meet on Sunday afternoon.

We met in the same conference room, amid telltale evidence of a late Saturday night staff meal of pizzas and sodas. I quickly removed empty food containers and unopened Diet Pepsis from the table and pushed the overflowing trash container into a corner. This time the only clinical staff at the meeting were myself, Dr. Rashid, and Jolene Hunter, her ICU nurse. The Maxwell family was well represented by Evie and Frank, Ellis and his wife, Ellis Jr., and Cici. In the past two days Evie and Ellis had been carefully updated regarding the changes in her neurological condition, the scans, the medications she had received, and her surgery. They knew that her prospects for recovery were now nonexistent.

After briefly reviewing the things that had been done to maintain her physical condition in the past week, I mentioned that, in addition to all the treatments, we were also doing a few things intended to comfort and honor Mrs. Maxwell.

Chaplains were seeing her every day and praying over her. Her own minister had visited twice—and was here now, having driven over after their congregation's Sunday service. Our No One Alone palliative care volunteers were also visiting daily and making sure that the CD player was working and that there was music playing in her room. A "Get to Know Me" poster was taped on a floor-to-ceiling sliding glass door that formed the wall between her room and the common space of the intensive care unit. On it her family had written that she likes to be called Maxie, and next to "occupation" had written, "the best baker and mother in the world." The rest was left blank except for at least a dozen photos of Maxie in happier times. She usually had an apron on in the pictures, often standing in a kitchen or behind a dinner table. There were holiday pictures and one of Elbert and her at a fair. In most pictures there were several children, most of whom were clearly unrelated. On an old photo that had been obliquely taped in place, she appeared to be in her forties and was sitting behind a much younger, trimmer Frank on a motorcycle, holding her son-in-law tightly as he grinned to the camera.

I had looked at every photo and now commented on the richness of their family life. "I can tell that she will be sorely missed," I said.

Frank piped up in a groan. "Doc, she is already missed," he said.

There was a moment's silence, and then Ellis Jr. laughed, which caused the rest of the family to giggle self-consciously. The medical professionals in the room sat quietly clueless until Evie explained the inside joke. Maxie was known to bake eight to ten pies for Thanksgiving dinner; there would be pumpkin and peach and two kinds of apple and coconut cream pies and at least one of Frank's favorite, a pecan–maple sugar pie. This Thanksgiving he had to settle for just apple and pumpkin and he had grinned and borne the hardship.

The moment's levity did not diminish the solemnity of our discussion. Though it was expressed with humor, Frank's statement expressed the stark fact that Maxie was irreplaceable. Things would never be nearly the same. In so many ways, she was already gone. They would still be a family connected in their shared loved of Maxie. Even the foster children she helped raise and friends who were not related to Maxie by blood or marriage would always share a bond of their love for her and how important she had been in their lives.

"When we last met, we had planned to come together again on Tuesday and I expected that we would have difficult decisions to make about how long to continue intensive treatments. As it happens, I think that the biology of her condition is now making those decisions for us." I paused before concluding, "It is fair to say that nature itself has declared that Mrs. Maxwell is dying."

In discussions of this sort, I use the word "nature" knowing that for religious people in the room, it may be heard as a synonym for God. That's okay. I only presume to talk about God with patients if I know what they believe. Otherwise, I usually ask them to tell me about their beliefs, if it would be helpful for me to know. In learning about their beliefs, traditions, and the language they use, I can often communicate with and support people in little ways that can mean a lot.

In that spirit and hope, I spoke softly to Cici. "I know that you have felt that God was looking after Maxie and that he had a plan. Do you think it is possible he is calling her home?"

"Yeah. I think Maxie is tired and she is ready to go to heaven," she said. Her expression was sad but composed. She was not angry and seemed resigned.

"So, I sense people here are in sad agreement that the time has come to allow Mrs. Maxwell to die." I paused and looked at each person in the room. Nods and eye contact affirmatives all around. Except for myself and Dr. Rashid, people were touching or hugging the person next to them.

"I want to assure you that she will not feel distress as the ventilator is stopped and endotrachial tube is removed. Her death will be gentle. We will medicate her with extra doses of pain medication and a sedative—and will be standing by if there is any hint of discomfort. Sometimes people live for minutes to a few hours after a ventilator is stopped, but in this particular situation, I expect she will die very quickly.

"We are not in a rush to do this. If you wish to take a few hours to have family or friends visit, please do."

Evie and Ellis both had a list of people whom they had notified and had been coming by throughout yesterday, last evening, and this morning. They felt that they would need only another few minutes at her bedside with her, once again, the center of the family. Their minister would say a few prayers. They did not want to be present when she died.

This meeting lasted just twenty minutes.

Forty-five minutes later, I accompanied Dr. Rashid during the procedure to withdraw the ventilator from Mrs. Maxwell. We had not worked together in this manner before. As a senior physician and as an educator, I wanted to make sure before proceeding that Dr. Rashid had a clear understanding of the procedures. He and I reviewed in detail what medications we would be giving, in what doses, and the sequence of steps we'd take in discontinuing the ventilation.

While Mrs. Maxwell's family and minister visited and prayed at her bedside, Dr. Rashid and I met with Jolene, her nurse, and a respiratory therapist outside her room. We discussed what we expected to occur and agreed on the doses of fentanyl, a narcotic pain medication, and midazolam, a Valium-like sedative, to use and made sure extra doses were immediately available if needed. Since family would not be in the room, we decided to leave the cardiac monitor on to follow the electrical activity of her heart, while turning the audible alarms off.

Her family left her room and headed for the waiting room.

As Dr. Rashid and I stood by, Jolene administered the medications and the respiratory therapist turned off the ventilator and disconnected the ventilator from Mrs. Maxwell's tracheostomy tube. She died peacefully. There was no hint of struggle, no grimace, twitch, or moan. The only perceptible change as the cardiac tracings went from a sinus rhythm at 86 beats per minute to asystole—no beats at all—was an abrupt change in her color from flesh pink to steel gray.

As Jolene cleared away now extraneous equipment from around Mrs. Maxwell's bed, Dr. Rashid and I went to the waiting room and informed Evie, Ellis, and the other members of her family that she had died peacefully. We invited them to spend time with her body if they wanted to do so.

3.

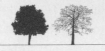

Balancing Acts—Weighing Potential Benefits Against Risks and Burdens

When my good friend Herb Maurer was diagnosed with a bad cancer, I knew he was likely to die of it—so did he. In the treatment decisions that lay ahead, I didn't want him *just palliated* (a phrase I detest when other doctors say it). Certainly, I expected and would make sure that expert attention was paid to Herb's comfort and quality of life. However, if there was a decision to be made at the moment, plainly and simply, I wanted him cured.

I remember the afternoon in March 2007 when he told me he was ill. I was walking down the carpeted central corridor of the medical center called Main Street. I thought I noticed Herb's distinctive hulking frame in the distance, lumbering toward me among the pedestrian stream. I was headed toward the cancer center on the ground floor and just approaching the rotunda, a large open area with a broad granite-countered octagonal information desk that sits directly below a pyramidal glass ceiling—the medical center's landmark architectural feature. It is an intersection that has the feel of a busy thoroughfare or mall. Main Street was sun-drenched that spring day.

"Herb, how are you? Haven't seen you in months," I said as we shook hands.

Herb Maurer was one of the smartest oncologists and most dedicated physicians I have ever known. He was prone to dress informally, but his jeans and flannel work shirt were a bit worn and torn, even for Herb.

He smiled wanly and said, "Well, I've got cancer," in a mockingly matter-of-fact tone.

"What? What kind of cancer? Tell me you're joking, right?"

We were standing in windowed sunshine, in the most public of places, with the medical center's professionals, outpatients, vendors, and visitors coursing around us.

"No, it's no joke. I got jaundiced over the weekend and went to the emergency department. They ran a screening panel and, sure enough, my LFTs [liver function tests] are up. A CT scan showed a mass at the common duct. I just came from Greg's office," he added, referring to Greg Ripple, an oncology colleague. "I figure I either have pancreatic cancer or a cholangiocarcinoma. I am betting on cholangio because I am also anemic." By the end of his explanation, his voice had assumed an academic tone, as he wondered aloud about an interesting detail of his own clinical presentation.

"I am headed right now to see Stu Gordon for an ERCP to have him biopsy this damn thing and see if he can place a stent," he said, his voice still slightly detached.

"Oh, shit, Herb," I said. "How are you holding up? How is Letha taking this news?" In addition to being husband and wife, Herb and Letha, who is also an oncologist, shared a busy medical practice in nearby Vermont.

"Well, it sucks. She's having a hard time, I think. We are just taking things one day at a time. I am likely going to need your services before too long. But for now, I am going to see what we can do. I'll need a PET-CT [positron emission tomography–computerized tomography] scan later this week and we'll see if there is any chance of getting this thing out."

I watched Herb head off to endoscopy for his ERCP, short for endoscopic retrograde cholangiopancreoscopy. The gastroenterologist, Dr. Stuart Gordon, would give him intravenous medications to relieve the pain and sedate him. Then, as Mr. Thorsen's gastroenterologist had done for him, Stuart would pass a flexible lighted scope through Herb's mouth and throat, down his esophagus to his stomach, and into his duodenum, the first part of the small intestine. Stuart would identify the opening (or ampula) from which bile from the liver and gallbladder and the digestive juices from the pancreas flowed into the duodenum. He would then thread a slender guide wire upstream (retrograde) into the duct system and pass a small plastic brush attached to another wire through the scope. Any cells that were collected on that brush would be sent to a pathologist who could examine them for evidence of cancer. Before removing the scope, if possible, Stuart would pass a short, thin metal stent over the guide wire and position it within the duct to keep bile draining into the duodenum.

The PET-CT scan Herb was scheduled to have later in the week is a combined scanning technique for revealing sites of metabolically active tumors in three dimensions corresponding to computerized images of a person's internal anatomy. In Herb's situation it was intended to find— or hopefully exclude—sites of metastatic cancer. If present, it would mean his cancer was Stage IV and that surgery was out of the question.

Even now, he knew well that prospects for surgery were slim. And yet surgery was the only chance he had of cure. He knew that, too. Today, there were no decisions to be made. But Herb knew that he would likely be wrestling with treatment options in the near future.

He was painfully aware that his chances of "getting this damn thing out," as he put it, were slim at best. Whether it was "cholangio" or pancreatic, very few people survive cancer in this region of the body. Those who do usually have their cancers found by accident, before the malignant growths have caused any symptoms and before they have spread, even microscopically. Nevertheless, Herb was determined to exert due diligence and hope for the best. It is what he would have done if he were the oncologist for a patient with the same condition. And as a faculty member of Dartmouth's Hematology-Oncology Fellowship program, it is what he had taught dozens of oncologists-in-training to do.

Herb became an oncologist before there was such a thing. Early in his career, after returning from a stint as an army physician in Vietnam, Herb gravitated toward treating people with cancer. When he started in practice the body of knowledge concerning cancer treatment had not yet earned specialty status. He absorbed the science of oncology like a sponge and seemed to intuitively understand the myriad ways cancer plays mischief—and wreaks havoc—with people's bodies. In addition to becoming a consummate clinician, Herb conducted early research in the treatment of lung cancer that pushed the forefront of the fight against the disease. And he was a driving force in founding the Norris Cotton Cancer Center at Dartmouth, where I now work.

But those descriptions barely begin to describe the man. Herb was multitalented, a man of strong beliefs—which he loudly voiced—on everything from the right treatments for lung cancer to national politics, from raising children to gourmet cooking, from furniture making to visual arts—and an irreverent, uproarious sense of humor. Having dinner with Herb and Letha would always stimulate and nurture my palate, mind, and soul.

He was an imposing figure. Herb's tall, muscular frame, bushy, full-curl, handlebar mustache, booming voice, and sartorial preference for checkered flannel shirts made for odd first impressions. Think Paul Bunyan meets Wilford Brimley. Herb tended to mumble, making him sound like a baritone with a mouthful of marbles and often making it hard to be sure what he was saying. When he asked a question that someone didn't understand, he would repeat it louder. Only occasionally did that help. When he was annoyed or impatient—which was not uncommon—his deep sonorous voice sounded like rolling thunder. Often you still couldn't be sure just what he was saying, but you knew he really meant it!

For all his bluster, there was not an unkind spicule of bone in Herb Maurer's body. Herb exuded warmth and most patients fell in love with him within the first ten minutes. His melodious mumbles and genuine concern melted people's fears (although I was never entirely certain they understood what he said). A hug from Herb could soothe a patient more than any medication ever made.

No wonder they bonded to him. On admission to the hospital people he cared for would proudly identify themselves to staff saying, "I am one of Dr. Maurer's patient's." The loyalty flowed both ways. Years after he and Letha had left the medical center to go into private practice together in a nearby town, Herb would show up on weekends, in a flannel shirt and snow boots, to make social visits to any of his patients who happened to be in our university hospital.

Actually, except for the outer coat he carried and sneakers he wore, he didn't look all that different that day at the rotunda.

"So, why don't you check in with me later in the week—or call Letha," Herb said. He was ready to move on. Our chance encounter had lasted barely two minutes, but I could sense that Herb wanted to stay focused on getting through his appointments and scan. The appointment he had to get to provided a good excuse to curtail our conversation before it got too sad or sentimental.

"Okay. Take care of yourself, will ya?" I said, not even knowing myself what I meant.

"Yeah." He waved to me as he headed off to the fourth floor.

It didn't seem real. As I walked on I realized I had just got a small dose of what Herb and Letha must have been feeling the past few days. It was disorienting. They must be emotionally reeling, I thought, trying their best to maintain, or regain, an even keel. His cancer had taken hold not just of his body, but of his and Letha's lives. I wondered what the best care was for Herb now and what it would entail in the future.

It is a basic tenet of medical ethics that, except in dire emergencies, consent from the person being treated is required before any treatment is administered. When the patient is an underage child, parents are the ones who consent. When the risks of a treatment are significant—such as surgery or radiation or chemotherapy—formal "informed consent" is required, which usually entails patients (parents or designated decision-makers) signing a consent form attesting that they understand and accept the risks of the procedure.

The usual analysis of risks and potential benefits is straightforward: imagine a simple balance scale, in which the risks and potential benefits are at either end of a plank, supported by a central fulcrum. In this idealized metaphor, the plank begins perfectly horizontal, representing equipoise in the decision-making process, absent prejudice or predilection on the parts of either physician or patient. Of course, every physician applies his or her own judgment before ever suggesting a treatment to a patient. Doctors are trained to go through a "risk-benefit analysis" in their own minds to see if the treatment is even worthy of consideration.

But as medical treatments for serious conditions have become more sophisticated—often more risky but also more effective—ethical guidelines have evolved to respond to real-world complexities.

Today best practice in informed consent requires a process called shared decision-making. As the term implies, shared decision-making entails the collaboration of physicians and patients to examine the risks and potential benefits of a proposed treatment, balanced against the risks and known burdens of treatment in the process of coming to a joint decision about a treatment plan. Although it seems almost self-evident that decisions should be reached in this manner, traditionally medical decisions were made primarily, if not solely, by doctors.

One of the pioneers of this new, collaborative approach to health care decision-making is James Weinstein, an orthopedic surgeon and health service researcher. In the early 1990s, Weinstein was a prominent spine surgeon who recognized that there were pros and cons to operative and nonoperative treatments for back pain, even when a discrete problem, such as a slipped disk, could be diagnosed. Although patients who had surgery might feel better faster, there were uncommon but very serious immediate perioperative risks. He also noticed that by three or six months, patients seemed to do fairly well in terms of pain and function whether they had had surgery or conservative treatments, including physical therapy. Dr. Weinstein felt it was incumbent on him to carefully explain the risks and potential benefits of back surgery, and for the final decision to be one that he and his patient shared. This process seemed intuitively sound and was warmly received by patients. Weinstein convinced his colleagues at DHMC's Spine Center to make this enhanced approach to informed consent standard practice.

Within the medical center, Jim Weinstein's approach gradually earned broad support. The Center for Shared Decision Making opened in 1998. Situated on Main Street, between the rotunda and the food court, the center is in a prime location that is intended to encourage walk-ins. There, people can find printed or video information about common surgeries, and treatments for cancer, lung and heart disease, kidney dialysis, and transplantations, and can receive one-on-one counseling if they wish. Someone who is healthy and considering whether to donate a kidney or portion of their liver to a relative or close friend can also find information or get questions answered at the center.

Nationally, Weinstein helped to establish the Foundation for Informed Medical Decision Making, which developed a series of evidence-based booklets and videos to fully inform patients who were considering whether or not to undergo tests or treatments for health problems for which there were no clearly right or wrong choices. The list of situations that the foundation addresses continues to expand: Whether to take hormone replacement therapy for menopausal symptoms? Whether to have a lumpectomy followed by radiation or a mastectomy if you're a woman who's been told you have early stage breast cancer? Whether to undergo a PSA (prostate-specific antigen) screening test for prostate cancer if you are a healthy fifty-year-old man? Whether to have radiation or a surgical prostatectomy if diagnosed with prostate cancer? In addition to cancer, there are materials on whether to treat your child's attention deficit disorder with medications, how to consider institutional versus home care for a parent with dementia, and on and on. All of this represents a dramatic shift from the way medicine has traditionally been practiced. In providing evidence-based guidance directly to patients and their families, the foundation and DHMC's Center for Shared Decision Making are advancing an important trend in health care for the twenty-first century.

In 2003 Jim Weinstein became the chair of the Department of Orthopedic Surgery. Under his stewardship, formal decision-making processes became part of the routine evaluation for back and spinal surgeries. He subsequently became director of The Dartmouth Institute for Health Policy and Clinical Practice, which advances decisional science and its application in practice, and in 2011 Weinstein became CEO and president of Dartmouth-Hitchcock Medical Center. It is fair to say that shared decision-making is well established within the ethos of the institution.

As an oncologist, Dr. Herb Mauer was already well-informed. And by temperament, there was never a doubt that Herb would be firmly in charge of decisions about what types and how much treatment he received. Yet, despite his many years of doctoring—or more likely *because of* his long clinical experience—he continually invited input and welcomed help from his doctors, friends, and family. Herb valued the expertise and wise perspective of his physician colleagues and did not make any major decisions without their considered opinions. Indeed, this collaborative approach had long been the way he practiced. In deciding whether or not to have any given treatment—and he had many—Herb spoke at length with Greg Ripple, his medical oncologist, and, depending on the specific treatment, with Bassim Zaki, his radiation oncologist, John Gemery, his interventional radiologist, and Stuart Gordon, his gastroenterologist. Also consistent with the way he practiced oncology, Herb wanted to be aggressive in treating his disease, but not foolish.

He knew the score—down to the details of every pitch. Ampullary carcinoma is highly life-threatening and very often lethal. It is actually slightly less lethal than either pancreatic cancer or bile duct cancer, each of which can cause identical symptoms and presentation. The only way to tell these different diseases apart is by looking at tumor cells under a microscope, conducting tests of serum biomarkers, and examining the genetic profile of the tumor.

People with cholangiocarcinoma, cancer that arises from bile duct cells, generally survive between two and a half and just over four years, depending on the size of the tumor, whether it has spread to lymph nodes or beyond, and whether there is microscopic infiltration of cancer cells into the outer lining of small nerves in the tissue surrounding the tumor. Larger tumors, those that have metastasized to lymph nodes or the liver or lungs, and those with perineural invasion all portend lower survival.

Within a week after being diagnosed—it turned out to be a cholangiocarcinoma as he'd suspected—Herb underwent a pancreoduodenectomy, a modified Whipple procedure. It was a big operation that typically requires months of recuperation as the gastrointestinal track adapts to the change in anatomy and digestion. But Herb sailed through surgery and recovered with remarkable speed. His indomitability seemed intact.

The surgery had removed all visible signs of cancer. The edges of the tissues removed—a portion of his duodenum, bile ducts, and pancreas—showed no signs of cancer under the pathologist's microscope. All of that was hopeful, but neither Herb nor his doctors thought that the cancer was gone. As soon as his wounds were healed, he decided to begin an aggressive course of chemotherapy, intended to kill or at least slow the growth of any remaining cancer cells.

Most cancer chemotherapy drugs are toxic to normal, healthy cells, particularly those that divide and reproduce often—such as cells lining the intestines, mouth, and hair follicles, and the blood-forming cells in bone marrow. Herb had been administering these agents—and more toxic earlier drugs—to cancer patients for years. He was all too aware of their side effects. Remarkably, however, Herb once again sailed through. Although his legendary appetite and digestion diminished for a while, and he lost a few pounds, he maintained his strength and for several months was even able to continue seeing patients two days a week.

Herb was passionate about life, which was why he fought so hard to preserve the lives of others. The lust for life that marked everything Herb did was undiminished by his illness; if anything, his illness increased his love of life. He was determined to use whatever time he had to live well—at least the time that wasn't conscripted to tests, outpatient treatments, or complications that landed him in the hospital.

In outward appearances Herb's overriding focus was fighting the cancer. He was not one to talk openly about his feelings or private thoughts. But as his friend and one of his physicians, I knew he was thinking about the broader, personal implications of his illness.

Roughly six weeks after his surgery, Herb asked me to see him clinically. He explained, "I am not there yet. But I'd have to be mighty lucky for this thing to go away, and I don't feel that lucky. You and your group are good at helping people through this. I want to make sure I don't overlook something that is important. I particularly want to do this right for Letha and my kids." He waved his hand in a gesture that telegraphed, "You know, the stuff you talk about in your books," before he said so aloud.

Despite his gruff, burly exterior, Herb was a physician who recognized the impact cancer has on the inner, tender, most personal aspects of people's lives. Whenever he referred patients to me he'd either buttonhole me at a Tumor Board meeting or call me up and tell me a bit about the person he wanted me to see before they made the appointment. Usually the people he referred had one or more complicated relationships and conflicts that were unresolved in their personal life.

A few patients subsequently told me that Herb had also suggested that they pick up *The Four Things That Matter Most*, a book I had written in which I talk about the value of people saying four things to one another before good-bye: Please forgive me. I forgive you. Thank you. I love you.

Now that he was ill, Herb took the advice to heart. With the same honesty that marked his treatment decisions, Herb had begun thinking about what would be left undone in his personal life if he died suddenly. He told me it was time to get around to things he had been putting off in the midst of a hectic professional life.

Herb had been married before and his first wife never forgave him for the separation. She remained angry with him through all these years and they had virtually no contact. Herb wanted to reach out to her, just to let her know that she still mattered to him.

They were parents of a son and daughter, now in their forties, whom Herb loved dearly. In recent years their mutually hectic lives made it hard to visit, and Herb felt he didn't see his older children and grandchildren nearly enough.

He and Letha also had children—three sons who were now young men scattered at colleges across the country and Scotland. His illness felt to Herb like a burden he would be imposing on all of them.

He brought up "the four things," so we started there.

"For sure," it would be good to say those things to each of his children, he said. However, his sense was that his first wife was still so angry with him that she would not sit still for such a conversation. He didn't think she would even tolerate him expressing his regrets and asking for forgiveness. I suggested he might write to her. In that way he'd be able to say what he wanted without the risk of heated emotions taking him off message.

We also talked about what he might expect in terms of a response from her. I reiterated a guideline I have been teaching for years: you can only be responsible for your side of any relationship. If, as Woody Allen observed, 80 percent of success is showing up, in situations of this nature, the other 20 percent involves arriving with good intentions. If our intentions are good and we are willing to ask for and offer forgiveness and express gratitude and loving feelings for another person, we usually feel better for having made the effort. Sometimes that needs to be enough. If the other person responds warmly, that's great. But, in matters of this sort, there is intrinsic value in making a good-faith effort. He said that all of this made sense and he would give it some thought.

I asked his thoughts on leaving a legacy for his children, grandchildren, and generations to come. Earlier in the spring, Letha and Herb had attended an evening public lecture at the medical center on the topic of ethical wills, hosted by our Palliative Care Service. The presenter, Dr. Barry Baines, is a palliative care physician from Minnesota who has been revitalizing the ancient tradition of ethical wills as a way for adults, especially parents, to write down bits of family history, things they think are most important, the values they hold highest, and special wisdom they want to leave to their children and future generations.

"Yes," he said, "Letha and I have talked about both of us setting aside time to do it."

In cancer of this sort, most victories tend to be short-lived. And so it was that Herb's cancer did recur, to his and all of our disappointment, but to no one's surprise.

Somehow, over the years he had integrated so much experience treating the disease that he had acquired a knack of thinking like different types of tumors. Perhaps because he had expected the cancer to return, he was prepared and able to maintain a problem-solving approach to each new obstruction to bile flow or bleeding that occurred.

Now more than ever Herb made full use of medical opportunities to extend his life and alleviate his discomfort. He was selective in choosing aggressive treatments. He took three rounds of potent chemotherapy. He had surgery to bypass an intestinal blockage. When he became jaundiced, he had endoscopic and radiology procedures to stent or re-stent clogged bile ducts or to control bleeding. In total, he underwent eighteen CAT (computerized axial tomography) scans and eight or more treatments.

Herb knew that every one of these interventions came with pain and risks of bleeding or infection. In fact, he ended up in the hospital on three occasions with fevers from bacteria in his blood after these procedures.

Through it all he never denied how seriously ill he was and how threatened his life was. Before any treatment decision, Herb would take stock; he, Letha, and his physicians would weigh the chances that the treatment would work against the discomfort and risk that it would bring. He would honestly discuss his current quality of life and whether it was worth sustaining. In Herb's case, for many months, the honest answer was yes.

Nevertheless, every time he was hospitalized, he made sure that there was a DNR order in his medical record. As much as he wanted to live, if his heart suddenly stopped, he wanted to die naturally. He didn't want anyone to perform CPR because he knew that even in the unlikely event that it restarted his heart, it would just mean that he would die in an ICU.

Despite weakness that forced him to nap most days and eventually to get around with a cane, Herb's quality of life remained well worth sustaining for over two years. Early on he had been able to work part-time, travel to see his children and their families, paint, and garden. Over time his energy and ability to do the things he most enjoyed took a stair step down with each new episode of biliary obstruction, bleeding, or infection and the corresponding percutaneous procedure and hospitalization. Whenever he felt stronger, he resumed chemotherapy, which may have extended his life, but also took a lot out of him. Each step was a new normal. He took things slow, adjusted his expectations, and relied more and more on Letha to get around.

For Herb, the process of balancing the potential benefits versus the risks and burdens of any proposed treatment rested on his current quality of life at this late stage of his illness. No cancer treatment could substantially improve his quality of life. He was already fighting just to hold steady against the downstream current. Each time a new complication occurred, a procedure could, at best, reestablish his most recent "new normal" life. In basing his decision-making on his running assessment of his own quality of life, it was as if the very ground on which Herb stood leaned either toward or away from a proposed treatment. This was a thoughtful and highly personal geometry. But in general he adapted and found ways of making his days worthwhile.

Eating was one way. Remarkably, until the last week of life, he had a pretty good appetite and thoroughly enjoyed each evening's meal. That meant a lot to Herb. Whenever we discussed one of the proposed treatments, he would comment on his appetite.

One morning, I visited Herb in the hospital. He had been admitted for another interventional radiology treatment, this one to cut off blood supply to part of the tumor in his liver. Herb told me, "I've been having *full meals*—from appetizers to desserts—and *enjoying them*." It was his way of literally bringing gut instinct to making decisions. The balance clearly tilted in the direction of preserving life.

On a Saturday evening a few weeks before he died, my wife, Yvonne, and I had dinner with Herb and Letha at their home. We started with oysters and gin and tonics, and then feasted on pizzas homemade by their son, Jason.

I remember thinking, once again, it all seemed so surreal. It was tragic, and yet there was a point during dinner when Herb looked at me with his head cocked, shoulders hunched, and brows arched, and I had to laugh. In that moment, with his innocent, quizzical expression and full-curl mustache he resembled Salvador Dalí against a backdrop of oysters on the half shell that looked a lot like Dalí's surrealistic melting watches.

When his lack of energy and increasing discomfort dragged his quality of life down and shifted the potential benefit-burden balance, Herb entered hospice care. He and Letha welcomed the help at home. For several weeks he held court as a virtual parade of people visited. On what turned out to be his last evening, Herb sat with his family, viewing hundreds of pictures of their lives together. The next morning, he felt too weak to get up and spent the day in bed. He was comfortable, except for an episode of losing his breath that required an injection of morphine followed by an injection of midazolam, emergency medications that our palliative care team and the hospice had in place. Thankfully, they worked to soothe his discomfort.

During the last hours of his life, Herb opened his eyes, smiled, and gave a "thumbs-up" to a good friend who had stopped by. His hospice nurse was there. He was surrounded by Letha, his children, his grandchildren, and close friends as he took his last breath.

It would be easy to lionize Herb, but it would not do him justice.

He was a brilliant, talented, funny, and warm human being. During his funeral and later at a memorial service held at the medical center, person after person told stories of Herb's intellect, compassion, humor, and quirks. People commented on his courage and integrity during the past two years. It was all true. But below his usually calm—fatalistic—demeanor, things were turbulent. He didn't take to illness and dying easily.

Herb's deeply personal, emotional struggles with his cancer are what make his deliberations about treatment—his negotiations about his diminished life, double-edged treatments, and death—so authentic and valuable as examples to me and others. He didn't embrace his illness—it still sucked—he merely accepted the reality of it and, of necessity, dealt with it. Herb's adaptation was not a New Age experience or any sort of spiritual transformation. It was Human Development 101. Herb saw his illness and dying as another crisis of life, something one could only try to avoid for so long. Ultimately, he had to face it and, if he could, grow through it.

Letha told me that Herb had sent his first wife a letter but had never heard back. She shrugged but added that Herb had said he'd felt better for having tried.

Faced with a situation that can break a person, shattering his or her sense of self and hope for the future, it is easy and almost seductive to succumb to suffering. When one's very body is literally eroding and one's world is falling apart, suffering exerts a gravitational pull. When personal annihilation awaits, it requires a conscious choice to avoid surrendering to depression and the depths of existential despair.

Herb's refusal to succumb was entirely consistent with his character. He chose to suck it up. His first priority remained the well-being of Letha and his children and extended family. Herb dealt honestly with the changes that his illness imposed. As a result, he lived through his illness and dying personally intact. He died well.

There is no universally right way for a person to die. What constitutes dying well for one person might be entirely wrong for another. The word "well" is both an adverb and an adjective. It can describe not only the dying process but, more important, the person who is dying. Herb was *well* as he was dying. Dying is the hardest, least desirable time in any of our lives. But it is possible to feel well within oneself and right with the world even as one dies. Therein lies hope for us all.

The costs of Herb's care during the thirty months from his diagnosis to death easily exceeded $250,000. Because Herb was older than sixty-five (he was sixty-eight when his cancer was diagnosed), Medicare paid for nearly all of it, including most of his medications.

As expensive as his final two years of life were, had he not continually balanced his love of life with his quality of life and desire to be at home with family at the end, it could have been much more expensive.

If Herb had decided to go back to the hospital on the morning he became sick for the last time rather than stay at home under Letha's and hospice care, he might well have lived a week or two longer, but would also likely have ended up in the ICU. The costs of those last days could have easily reached another $100,000.

From their perspective, Herb and Letha were simply carefully employing available medical treatments to make the best of a bad situation. The best care possible for Herb meant carefully applying medical science and technology to stem the tide of his cancer.

AS IT HAPPENED, during the last months of Herb's life I had participated in a conference on public policy related to end-of-life care. After the conference, a health journalist spoke with me concerning a magazine article she was working on about the "economics of dying." She asked my thoughts about for-profit medicine, overtreatment, the effects the high costs of end-of-life care have on other social programs, and, of course, rationing of health care.

It was a lively discussion. She said that she wanted to talk to a patient who was clearly dying but continuing to receive treatment that was exceedingly expensive. She was looking for one or more examples of egregious treatment that just might be motivated not only by concern for patients but also by some self-serving gain on the part of the treating physicians or their medical institution—if not financial, perhaps in the currency of reputation.

I told her that as much as I would like to help, that was not where I thought the story lay. I explained that I see a spectrum of people with serious conditions who, most bluntly, do not want to be dead. They have doctors who do not want their patients to die. And those doctors have an impressive array of technology for keeping people alive. All of this results in a continuum of decisions and treatments ranging from courageous and wise to foolhardy, and clinical outcomes that range from miraculous to macabre.

I told her about a fifty-seven-year-old man, who had been referred to our palliative care team by the liver transplant service. From reviewing his chart I knew that, much like Herb Maurer, Aaron Kramer had felt fine until he developed jaundice. Unlike Herb, Mr. Kramer's diagnosis was advanced cirrhosis, the result of a previously unsuspected hepatitis C infection that he had presumably acquired from briefly using IV drugs when he was in the military in his early twenties. He had unknowingly been harboring the "hep C" virus for years, as it silently inflamed and destroyed his liver.

Like both Herb and Gerry Thorsen, as soon as his jaundice was discovered, he underwent a slew of tests. When the hep C infection was found, the hepatologists—or liver specialists—at Dartmouth-Hitchcock started him on a combination of antiviral medications. For the first four months, he seemed to improve, but on routine follow-up testing, his serum level of alpha-fetoprotein was elevated, which is worrisome, since people with cirrhosis are at high risk to develop hepatocellular carcinoma. Sure enough, an MRI of his liver revealed two small tumors, highly suspicious for this primary liver cancer.

During a procedure by the interventional radiology team, one of the tumors was biopsied through a long thin needle that was passed just under his right ribs. A cytopathologist was on-site to look at the biopsy specimen under a microscope and confirmed the diagnosis of hepatocellular carcinoma or HCC. The two liver tumors were then destroyed by using radio frequency delivered through a needlelike probe that heated and killed the cancerous tissue.

Radio frequency ablation—or RFA—is an effective, often life-prolonging treatment for hepatocellular carcinoma. But it does not cure the disease. Once one locus of hepatocellular carcinoma occurs, it is a signal that others will almost inevitably follow. Most often, the new tumors are not true metastases. Instead of cells spreading from the original tumors to other portions of the liver, most are thought to be the same cell type of cancer that forms in different parts of the diseased liver, somewhat like a single strain of aggressive weed sprouting here and there in unfortunately fertile soil.

The only definitive cure for hepatocellular carcinoma is a liver transplant. But for someone with hepatitis C, after a successful transplant the virus reinfects the new liver and, even with antiviral medications, within a handful of years causes cirrhosis and, eventually, liver failure once again.

Still, for those lucky enough to receive a new liver, there is a 70 percent chance of living at least three years, and almost 60 percent of liver transplant recipients are alive fifteen years later. That is a stunning success rate for a uniformly fatal condition.

Of course, not everyone is that fortunate. About fourteen thousand people in the United States are on a waiting list for a liver transplant. (The median wait for a liver is just under a year nationally but varies regionally.) More than one in ten people will die before receiving a new liver. And at least another one in twenty leave the waiting list within six months. Many thousands of patients with liver disease never try to become "listed" because the evaluation process itself is so hard or because their condition makes them ineligible.

The hepatologists and oncologists in the Liver Failure clinic at DHMC wanted our team to help Mr. Kramer in adjusting to this difficult diagnosis, clarifying his goals for care and assisting in making decisions in the months ahead.

When we met Mr. Kramer he was still reeling from the latest bit of bad news. He had been hoping for a transplant but developed a suspicious lesion in his left lung. The day we met, his biopsy results had come back and, as feared, confirmed that the lung lesion was a metastasis. A liver transplant was now out of the question, since even one lung lesion was proof positive that there were other microscopic deposits of cancer lurking elsewhere. Even with a new liver, the disease was certain to recur somewhere.

He would now surely die of his disease. There were still some treatment options that could possibly slow the progression of the cancer—and Mr. Kramer's oncologist at DHMC started him on sorafenib (Nexavar), which had recently been FDA approved for treatment of this disease. In clinical trials it has been shown to modestly extend the lives of liver cancer patients (by 2.8 months) and costs between $6,600 and $8,600 a month, not counting routine laboratory tests and physician office visits.

The health journalist was intrigued and wanted to interview the patient I had described. (Of course, I had not told her his name.) I gave Aaron Kramer a call and he readily agreed to be interviewed. Two days later they met and spoke for over an hour via Skype.

Early that evening she e-mailed me and we spoke by phone. She said that they had a fascinating conversation but that she didn't think he fit for her article.

"Why not?" I asked. He was a dying person who was receiving exceedingly expensive treatments. She explained that during the interview he looked thin but fairly normal. He spoke about his current life, including his two daughters in graduate school, his horses—he is still able to ride—and the writing he was doing on a collection of essays he was trying to finish.

"Well, I've been looking for someone who is receiving exorbitantly expensive treatments for no good reason. Mr. Kramer explained his condition and treatments and, frankly, it all seems reasonable," she replied.

"Ahhh," I said, laughing out loud. "Let me get this straight: You have just interviewed a gentleman who has a uniformly lethal form of cancer that has already metastasized to his lung. He has been on a transplant list but has been removed because of the metastasis. His prognosis is poor. If I were still a hospice medical director, and Mr. Kramer wanted hospice care, I would sign him up for hospice care without hesitation. Instead, he is pursuing high-risk, quasi-experimental treatments at a cost of nearly

$75,000 per year. And you have decided that you think what he is doing is reasonable! Right?"

She was taken aback and silent. But I wasn't trying to be argumentative, so I continued.

"The fact is, I agree with you! What he is doing feels reasonable. All I can say is: welcome to my world. For what it's worth, I think Aaron Kramer is an ideal person for you to interview. His story epitomizes many Americans' experiences."

The truth is that if you are seriously ill but can still enjoy the time you have left, and a treatment that isn't all that toxic might help you live longer, why not try it?

On the other far end of the quality-of-life spectrum, if you are suffering terribly, endlessly, and there is an operation, a medical device, or a course of chemotherapy that offers real hope of greatly improving whatever life you have left—even if the treatment was dangerous and very expensive—it might seem worth the risk and costs.

And sometimes it is.

By all accounts Holly Block, a forty-three-year-old high school math teacher from Vermont, was the most loving, generous, and genuinely innocent person that people in her town ever knew. A petite, red-haired, freckled woman, she was dying from advanced cancer, but that was not the worst of her problems. A metastatic tumor pressing on her spine was causing "10 out of 10" pain and unrelenting suffering. Holly wasn't writhing with pain; instead, she held herself stone stiff, like a terrified novice on a tightrope, because almost any motion might set off another lightning bolt in her spinal cord.

Hell for Holly was not beyond this life; she was living in it. High doses of IV pain medication and steroids made her more comfortable, but groggy and constipated. We raised the possibility of neurosurgery, which carried risks of permanent paralysis but real hope of comfort. The operation would not help her live longer, but it would likely make her life less awful and that, for Holly, was worth any risk and price. Her reasons were quite different from Aaron Kramer's—he wanted life at any cost and she wanted relief, even if the cost was life—but in both cases the decisional landscape tilted in favor of treatment.

Dr. Perry Ball, a neurosurgeon at DHMC who specializes in spinal disorders, met Holly, studied her records and MRI, and agreed to consider the procedure. He is never eager to perform these operations. In spinal surgery of this nature, the nerve tracts that are being cut cannot be seen directly; their precise location can only be inferred from the surface anatomy of the spinal cord. Where to make a incision is a highly sophisticated estimation. Dr. Ball met with her and her husband and discussed the risks at length. He emphasized that this was a "destructive procedure" and that, unlike starting on a new medication, there is no way to undo the effects. There was a 5 to 10 percent chance of injuring motor nerves, rendering her unable to walk or even move her legs. There was about a 10 percent chance that the surgery would not alleviate her pain.

They listened carefully. Holly and her husband only had to consider the decision for a few minutes before announcing that they wanted to proceed—as soon as possible. She had surgery the following evening.

On rounds the morning after the four-hour operation, Holly smiled broadly as we entered her room. The deep "gnawing," "boring" pain in her pelvis and burning in her perineum were gone. She could move her legs and feet, even if she couldn't feel them. When I asked how she felt, she replied simply, "Safe at last."

Holly's predicament reveals the power of palliative care to apply sophisticated treatments, including highly technical procedures, in service of comfort and quality of life in our final months.

If only all decisions were sound and all outcomes were what people had hoped for. The result of Mrs. Maxwell's many treatments was far from what anyone in her family wanted. And few people would want to die the way Mr. Stephen Rollins did.

Stephen Rollins was a seventy-one-year-old man with diabetes and severe congestive heart failure with related, secondary liver and kidney problems. He was hospitalized with deep vein thrombophlebitis, or new blood clots, in his legs. The Critical Care Service asked our team to become involved when Mr. Rollins's blood pressure was dangerously low and he was requiring pressor medications in the ICU. The active coagulation that resulted in the clots had consumed all his clotting factors; therefore, paradoxically, he was now bleeding from any place on his body that he had had an IV or blood test taken.

Mr. Rollins had long been adamant that he wanted a heart transplant. When I met him, Mr. Rollins appeared ill. He said he was exhausted and sleepy from pain and anxiety medications. I asked him if he would impose any limits on treatments he was given at this time. Specifically, I asked him whether he wanted to have CPR performed if his heart stopped, and he said, "Yes!" After I dutifully explained that CPR would not likely work if his heart stopped beating effectively or his blood pressure couldn't be kept high enough to circulate oxygen throughout his body, and he said, *"Yes!"* again, more loudly. His daughter who was present for our conversation and seemed annoyed by my questions, explained, "Steve Rollins doesn't have quit in him."

In listening to the story of his life, I quickly came to realize that this never-say-die attitude was a lifelong characteristic, part of the warp and woof of Steve Rollins. It had served him well through previous illnesses and hardships, including the death of his wife and a brother, and a fire that destroyed his business. He was a model of perseverance for many people who knew and loved him.

Mr. Rollins didn't have quit in him, but his predicament was akin to someone in the pre–Wright brothers era whose efforts to fly were captured in those grainy, silent newsreels. Earnestly, courageously, they ran off cliffs or leapt from platforms, flapping the wings of devices that they hoped would keep them aloft, only to plummet to ground. For people with advanced, incurable conditions, mortality is a bit like gravity. Ultimately, it is the *force majeure* and will have its way with them, and us all. As a physician, in addition to helping people live as long and as well as possible, I can help people with advanced illness live with the fact of mortality and soften their final descent.

Sometimes, in situations of this sort, the most helpful and compassionate thing I can do is to say gently, but without equivocating, "I am sorry, but whatever we do at this point, you are dying." Similarly, to the family of a seriously ill person, sometimes plainly stating, "Your father is dying," can be a gift in the most difficult of times.

These are hard things for anyone to hear. Seasoned physicians know that news of this nature is best delivered when seated with the ill person or their family in a quiet and private place. It is not something to be said in a waiting room or hospital hallway.

Experienced physicians also know that a high degree of trust is needed for such a statement to be accepted. When I was growing up in the 1950s and 1960s, if a doctor said, "Your father is dying," it was like nature itself had spoken. The doctor was not communicating a decision or even an opinion; he was simply stating a fact, making plain something that, from his technical expertise, he knew to be true. Despite the sadness it evoked, the unequivocal quality of the news allowed people to prepare for what lay ahead.

I am not nostalgic for this era of medical practice. At that time, "shared decision-making" happened when the doctor shared his decision with his patient. Still, I wish it were easier these days for physicians to shoulder more of the weight of decisions that can be crushing for patients and families to bear alone.

In America's hospitals today, instead of being accepted as a statement of fact, a doctor saying "Your father is dying" can be heard by a family as an accusation. A physician who is not sensitive to the level of trust—or distrust—people have, or their readiness to accept such bitter truths, risks having his or her pronouncement challenged. At worst, the statement can be misconstrued as an unholy attempt to withhold expensive, lifesaving treatments. In this way, a doctor's well-meaning attempt to lift a weight from people's shoulders can backfire, destroying therapeutic trust with the very people he or she seeks to serve.

Trust is a rare commodity in health care today. Doctors tend to know their patients less long and less well than in earlier times. Today, there are myriad specialists and complex treatments to consider. And nearly every week, the headlines carry a story of someone whose life was saved by a treatment that did not exist a few years or even months ago, reinforcing hopes that with the *right* specialist and treatments at the *right* medical center, death can be forestalled.

Uncertainty underlies much of the stress and anxiety associated with making decisions about medical treatments. Even though death is dreaded, naming what is occurring as "dying" sweeps away uncertainty and places any pending decisions in a clear context. When a family is able to acknowledge that the person they love is dying, any family tensions regarding treatment decisions tend to dissolve. At such times, within a family's inevitable sadness, it is often possible to detect a sense of relief.

I only make dire statements about an individual's life expectancy when I am thoroughly confident that I am describing the person's condition rather than opining about how long a person might live. When maximal disease treatments are becoming increasingly ineffectual and the person is approaching death, I may say, "Biology is taking the decisions we have been wrestling with out of all of our hands."

I said words of that sort to Mrs. Maxwell's family as she lay in the ICU dying from a series of strokes caused by emboli from an infected heart valve.

Being concrete and unequivocal can be a gift, but it is a gift that not all families are willing to accept. When a patient or family member cannot accept—or even acknowledge—that dying is happening, such counseling can fall flat. When someone is dying, certainty brings clarity, but also acute emotional pain. People may cling to uncertainty because it preserves hope for a longer life and prevents—or at least delays—the stabbing, searing pain of grief.

In what seems like a desperate attempt to avoid that pain, sometimes families interpret any greater-than-zero prognosis as good news. I have heard a doctor tell the family of a gravely ill ninety-two-year-old man who was in cardiogenic shock and being kept alive (barely) with a ventilator and intravenous pressors that there was less than a one in a hundred chance of him surviving. That was enough for his children and grandchildren who hoped for his recovery to instruct the doctor to press on. His son, who was nearly seventy, explained, "You don't know my dad. He survived being shot down over Europe and a German prison camp. He can get through this, too."

Doctors who push back, labeling such reasoning as unrealistic, may find that anger is the next defense against grief. Over many years, I learned this the hard way. "Who are you to render this opinion?" "What are your credentials?" "Why are you saying this and not the other specialists?"

The pointed questions were aimed at me but were intended to undermine not merely my credibility but certainty itself. The aggrieved individual may go elsewhere seeking a second, third, or fourth opinion with doctors in Boston, New York, or Rochester, Minnesota. Questing for the right specialists or hospitals can be savvy advocacy, but it can also be a way of keeping uncertainty alive into the future.

Without sufficient trust, I am left to listen, acknowledge the family's concerns, and acknowledge the fact that nobody can know with absolute certainty how long a person will live. If they are willing to listen, I can offer to explain why I believe the person they love is dying. I can answer each and every question as fully as possible and offer to communicate with doctors of their choice in other centers. In my commitment to serve patients and their families, it seems the least I can do. At times, it is the most I can do—or rather, the most that a family will allow me to do.

Anger is a way of holding sadness at bay; the emotions are two sides of the same coin. Anger is energizing. When we are angry we look out, adopt a protective posture, and get ready for action. In contrast, sadness saps our energy. When sad, we look inward, become reflective, and are aware of our vulnerability. When someone is dying, becoming angry— with the disease or treatments, or the doctors and hospitals—may be what a grieving person needs to do for his or her own emotional well-being. Even if the anger is irrational, for a brief time it can be adaptive. Although it never feels good to be the target of a family member's anger, when it happens to me I try not to take it personally. If being angry at me can temporarily help people with the pain of learning that they are dying, or that a father or mother, brother or sister, son or daughter is dying, so be it. But I certainly don't relish their anger and I don't want to add to any patient's or family's distress. So I try to convey the news as sensitively as I can, when people are able to hear it.

In Mr. Rollins's case, our team and I never were able to develop much rapport with him or his family. I was unable to even offer to bear that load. In our consultation we described his and his family's goals of care as "all treatments possible." Within a day of meeting them, Mr. Rollins became too ill to engage in conversation and his family never perceived that there were decisions to be made. He developed acidosis from toxins building up in his bloodstream and was intubated and mechanically ventilated to maintain oxygenation. His hands were covered in padded cotton mittens to keep him from inadvertently dislodging his endotracheal tube and the IV tubing and wires connecting him to medication pumps and monitors. After his blood pressure dropped, despite maximal doses of pressor medications, he developed electromechanical dissociation—signifying that there were electrical waves on the EKG (electrocardiogram) monitor but no pulse or effective contractions of his heart. CPR was briefly performed and he was pronounced dead.

Steve Rollins never quit and never said die, but mortality still had its way.

Three weeks after he died, I received a handwritten note from Mr. Rollins's daughter. She said that she felt her father got good care, but only because they had pushed for it. She wrote that I had been heavy-handed in pressuring him to make decisions to die against his will.

Part Three

Palliative Care: Completing the Therapeutic Continuum

4.

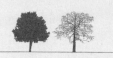

Palliative Care—
A Surprising New Specialty
(Hint: It's Not Just for Dying)

O f course I will talk with her, Dr. Byock. And you know what I am going to tell her? I'll tell her you people gave me my Mickey back!" It was mid-January 2007. I called Sandy Zimble to ask if she would be willing to talk with a journalist about the palliative care and hospice that she and her husband, Mickey, experienced.

Earlier in the day, Reed Abelson, a health reporter for the *New York Times*, had interviewed me for a story she was writing about the growth of specialized palliative care teams in leading American hospitals. Hospital-based palliative care was still quite new. Palliative care had grown out of hospice care in the United States and the medical component, palliative medicine, had formally earned status as a subspecialty in September 2006. Reed had asked how our program receives referrals, how receptive other doctors are to the palliative care team being involved, and whether willingness to consult us varies among specialties. I filled her in on the ways our team was becoming increasingly integrated within expanded multispecialty health care teams treating people with serious cancers, heart disease, and liver disease, as well as people with multisystem organ failure in the ICUs.

About twenty minutes into our conversation, Reed abruptly changed the subject.

"Did you read Art Buchwald's book?" she asked. "If so, what did you think of it?"

Art Buchwald had recently died at his son's home in Washington, D.C. Late in 2006, the celebrated humorist and columnist for publications such as the *Paris Review, Herald Tribune, Washington Post*, and *Newsweek* had published *Too Soon to Say Goodbye*, a memoir of his life after becoming a patient in a hospice facility the previous February. Having been a fan of his columns and books over the years, I picked up a copy shortly after the book came out and enjoyed it thoroughly. Typical of Buchwald, his book was insightful, self-deprecating, and funny.

In *Too Soon to Say Goodbye*, Buchwald writes about how he came to be admitted to a hospice facility in the Washington, D.C., area. His kidneys had shut down, but he didn't want dialysis. He had advanced peripheral vascular disease—and was very likely facing the amputation of one leg. He didn't want that either. He checked in to the hospice fully expecting that he was dying, but instead, his kidneys started working enough to keep him alive. He recounts visits he received from dignitaries and literati from around the world during the five months he spent in the hospice residence. Even in his dying he didn't take himself too seriously. He dreams about a big funeral and conspires to get an obituary in the *New York Times*.

Buchwald thrived in the hospice residence and was eventually discharged in June 2006. He spent the summer and fall at his home on Martha's Vineyard where he wrote *Too Soon to Say Goodbye*, all the while continuing to visit with family and friends, inevitably saying his own good-byes. In his book and during a number of interviews he gave while at the hospice facility and in subsequent months, Buchwald credited the care he received for giving him the chance to get better and live longer.

Reed Abelson asked me how often people live longer than expected with hospice care. At the time, I didn't have statistics I could report to her. However, I told her that in my experience it was fairly common.

"After all," I asserted, "although we work in hospice and palliative care, we are doctors and nurses. We are not specialists in dying as much as specialists in taking care of people who are seriously ill and may die. In taking good care of people with advanced diseases—making sure they are physically comfortable, eating and drinking, 'pooping and pee-ing,' sleeping and getting around as well as possible—it is not all that surprising that they live a bit longer. Occasionally, some of our patients, such as Art Buchwald, live *quite a bit* longer."

For instance, I explained, we help a lot of people with advanced cancer to tolerate treatments that are effective against their tumors but have difficult side effects. In alleviating their symptoms and optimizing their ability to eat and drink, be active and rest, people with cancer are able to stay in the fight longer. If a time comes when chemotherapy and radiation prove more toxic than therapeutic, we can still help people live as well and as long as possible. Patients with late-stage cancers commonly find that when they are finally free of the side effects of treatment, they feel better and stronger. In *living with*, rather than relentlessly fighting their cancer, they ultimately live longer.

Reed was intrigued. "I can see that," she said and then asked, "Can I talk to one of those patients or their families?"

"Yes, I think so," I said. "Let me make a phone call or two and I'll get back to you."

I gave the matter some thought and then called the Zimbles.

I had met Sandy and Mickey Zimble in June 2006 (about the time Buchwald was headed to Martha's Vineyard). Mickey had been admitted to the inpatient cancer unit at Dartmouth-Hitchcock Medical Center four days earlier because of severe abdominal pain and profound weakness. His oncologist, Dr. Ernstoff, asked our team to help with his pain and assist him and his wife in coping with the regrettable likelihood that he was dying.

Mickey managed to be friendly, but it was clear that he had no energy and little patience for conversation. He answered direct questions when he could.

"Where does it hurt?"

"Here," pointing to his right side.

"How many times did you move your bowels yesterday?"

"Two, I think."

But he often shrugged or said "I don't know," or looked to his wife, Sandy, to answer. And she did, often speaking for them both. For the first couple of days I knew them, Mickey mostly moaned as waves of abdominal cramps rumbled and, at times, roared within him.

He was no stranger to cancer. Mickey had had prostate cancer since 1995 and was initially treated with radiation and hormone therapy. He developed breast cancer in 1999 and had a mastectomy with negative lymph nodes, meaning there was no evidence the cancer had then spread. And he had a small, early-stage melanoma removed from his upper back in 2005. In early 2006 on the basis of a rising PSA, which indicated a likely recurrence of prostate cancer, he underwent treatment with a combination of anticancer drugs. Now, however, he was admitted with newly discovered liver tumors. This is not a usual pattern of prostate cancer. Indeed, biopsies of his liver lesions showed a high-grade neuroendocrine tumor—yet another cancer, which had possibly arisen from a biological transformation of his prostate cancer.

It was unlikely that he would dodge the bullet this time. His liver was swollen and tender to the touch. His right lower abdomen hurt worse, though there was nothing felt on physical examination or seen in that region on CT scans. With medication for pain, Mickey was reasonably comfortable, except for a few times an hour when he doubled over in paroxysms of intestinal spasm, which lasted two to three minutes.

The oncology team had started a low dose of intravenous morphine by PCA—patient-controlled analgesia—which gave him a button to push to administer an extra, metered dose of morphine when he needed it. The morphine worked but made him sleepy and mildly confused. He was also anxious, especially at night, which made it difficult for him to sleep. The lorazepam (Ativan) that the team had prescribed made him sleepy, at least for an hour or two, but left him more confused during the night and next day, which heightened his anxiety. The best thing for his nocturnal nerves was having Sandy stay with him overnight in a recliner in his hospital room.

On one of my visits to his room, I noticed a family photo album that Sandy had brought to the hospital. With her permission, I flipped through it and saw photos of Mickey in 1953, a young man of twenty-two at Cushing Academy. Handsome with thick, dark hair, neatly combed in a wave, and an intelligent, winning smile, he was preppy as could be in a crisply pressed shirt and blazer. Through the chronology of images of his college years, their early relationship, and into midlife, Mickey remained dashingly attractive. He became a self-made success in the scrap metal business, and he and Sandy raised a family. And he was dashing still as his hair turned silver and he retired to play golf and enjoy his children and grandchildren. But after surviving three bouts of cancer, and struggling against a fourth, Mickey was a shadow of his former self.

Our team got busy on several fronts, yet our contributions to Mickey's care were prosaic. There was nothing particularly dramatic to do—no diagnostic coup or dramatic procedure to perform or treatment to start. Palliative care for Mickey was merely mundane meticulous medicine.

We were interested in the details of his pain—how often it came, whether it was crampy or sharp, and whether he also felt an urge to defecate when it came. Similarly, we asked about his appetite—or lack of same—and what he was eating, plus how often he drank milk or ate dairy products, and so forth. Each of these questions helped us gain a sense of the possible physiology underlying his symptoms.

Another member of our team, Dr. Brill Jacobs, spent two hours with Mickey and Sandy during the initial palliative care consultation. She made specific recommendations for changes in his medications—using

a low continuous dose of fentanyl, another pain medication, and scheduled low doses of haloperidol for anxiety and confusion. Because he had
cramps and loose stools, she ordered a stool sample to be sent to the
laboratory and tested for "C. Diff," formally *Clostridium difficile*, a bacteria species that all too commonly causes diarrhea among debilitated,
hospitalized patients.

The next day, with the new medications, Mr. Zimble was a little better overall. His pain had slightly lessened, but he now had full-blown
diarrhea. Not surprisingly, the C. Diff test was positive. We started
him on metronidazole, one of the very few antibiotics effective against
the *Clostridium difficile* germ. Unfortunately, metronidazole commonly
causes side effects of its own, specifically nausea and an upset stomach,
and Mickey was no exception. It was another instance in which the treatment for a complication of a disease caused its own complications.

Over the next week, with our dogged clinical attention to his various diagnoses, doses of medications, and side effects, Mickey gradually
improved. In fact, on morning rounds of the eighth day of our team's
involvement in his care, when I saw Mickey in his hospital room, he was
up, sitting in a chair, and dressed in madras golf shorts, a pale green polo
shirt, and a tan sweater. He was more talkative than at any time since our
team had met him. He reported having a good appetite and said that he
had eaten most of his breakfast. He opined—really more announced—
that it was time for him to go home.

I was all for that. It was great to see him feeling so much better.
Going home was definitely possible, but it would take some preparation. Though markedly diminished, he still had mild diarrhea. He was
still weak on his feet, a "one person assist" in getting from bed to a chair
or to the bathroom. He still had a urinary catheter. He still had large
tumors in his liver. He was anemic. He was taking six different scheduled
medications—some once a day, some twice a day, and some three times
a day—and had four medications to use as needed for breakthrough
pain, nausea, anxiety, and sleeplessness.

As much as I wanted to help Mickey get home, I didn't want Sandy and him to run into problems at home that forced him to come back to the hospital, at least not if we could prevent them. That would feel like failure to Mickey and would be even more frustrating than waiting another day or two before going home.

I spent a long time that morning discussing hospice care with Sandy and Mickey. I explained that I thought it would be important for them to have the services that the local hospice program could provide. They knew that hospice cared for people who were dying and, while not surprised, were somber in realizing that Mickey now officially qualified as "dying." I explained that hospice is the most comprehensive program of care for people who were facing the end of life—and for their families. I explained that a nurse who specialized in hospice care would be assigned to them and while they would see that nurse most frequently, hospice care entailed a team—very much like our palliative care team, which they had come to know—with a physician, chaplain, social worker, and even volunteer visitors. Any or all of these components of the team at some point might be of help. Additionally, a physical therapist from hospice could see him at home and teach them both ways of keeping him active, exercising, and safe. Importantly, a hospice nurse would be available by phone and able, if needed, to make an urgent home visit any time of the day or night. A hospice physician was always on call and available in an emergency. Accepting hospice care meant that anti-cancer treatments would not be part of the plan. This is often a sticking point for patients. In Mickey's case, since Dr. Ernstoff clearly said he was too sick to receive more chemotherapy, that stipulation made little difference. For many people it does.

The very words "hospice" and "palliative care" tend to scare people. Although people who are struggling with cancer, heart disease, lung disease, or liver disease clearly benefit from the services that hospice and palliative care provide, for some the terms carry fearful symbolic power, even superstition. When I introduced myself as "Dr. Byock, from the Palliative Care Service" to Mr. Stamford, who was hospitalized for advanced heart failure, he responded defiantly, "I'm not that far gone!" The same week, another patient reacted to my suggestion that hospice would be helpful in her care and in supporting her family at home by plaintively asking, "Is there really no hope?"

Unfortunately, many people think accepting hospice—and by extension palliative care—means you have to give up on living and embrace your dying. It is a misconception that is rooted in Medicare regulations. Indeed, what is sometimes mistaken for "hospice philosophy" is actually a set of rules imposed by Medicare (as well as Medicaid and many insurance policies) that effectively requires people to choose between expensive disease-treatments and hospice care. No wonder they resist it.

This federal law passed in 1981 that established the Medicare benefit for hospice care restricted eligibility to people who had a life expectancy of six months or less, "if the disease runs its natural course." Someone covered by Medicare who is seriously ill is required to sign a hospice election form, indicating "full understanding of the palliative rather than the curative nature of hospice care as it relates to the individual's terminal illness."

Under the law, Medicare reimburses hospice programs at a fixed daily rate to provide home-based services that are "reasonable and necessary for the palliation or management of the terminal illness as well as related conditions." In return, hospice programs assume responsibility for all the costs of care associated with the terminal diagnosis.

Thus, if a seventy-five-year-old hospice patient with advanced lung cancer is admitted to the hospital with respiratory failure and dies after three days, his bill for upward of $27,000 would belong to the hospice program. If he lived a week or more, because he or his family decided to call 911 when he suffered breathlessness and in the emergency department he was intubated and sent to the ICU on a ventilator, that bill could run to over $100,000. Such charges can easily bankrupt a hospice program.

So it is not out of stinginess, but rather out of sound management and programmatic survival, that hospice organizations have been reticent to admit—and assume the financial responsibility for the care of—patients who are seeking active treatment for their disease. This explains, but does not excuse, why some hospice programs counsel patients to forgo treatments that might well benefit them. I am not talking about major surgery or highly emetogenic (translated: "makes you puke") chemotherapy, but merely a transfusion every few weeks for a woman with bone marrow failure, who is comfortable and able to enjoy her days but too anemic to get to the dining room, or a liter of intravenous saline every other day for a man with cancer and chronic diarrhea after extensive bowel surgery who is too dehydrated to sit upright without passing out.

On several occasions, I have had hospice programs refuse to admit patients I have referred because they were "not hospice appropriate" or "not ready for hospice," meaning that they might want to be hospitalized if they got an infection or, like the patients just mentioned, needed occasional blood transfusions or IV saline. At such times, I point out that the sharp division between life-prolonging and hospice care—the either-or choice—is not embedded in philosophy, clinical principles, or ethics but merely in statute. The Medicare regulations don't prohibit such treatments. They merely require the hospice to pay for them. That's a challenge particularly for smaller rural programs. However, many programs do provide these services despite the costs. When treatments like IV fluids or transfusions are feasible to provide and therapeutically meaningful to improving people's quality of life, they can be given as part of hospice care.

In fact, although Medicare's limitations have been encrusted in federal law, many private insurers, including a majority of Blue Cross Blue Shield companies, offer concurrent disease treatments and palliative care, including home hospice care, to people with serious, life-limiting conditions. Even before the 2010 health care reform act passed, United

Healthcare and Aetna were offering concurrent care to a segment of their clients.

The either-or choice between disease treatment and hospice care that Medicare imposes makes people equate hospice with "giving up." It's the main reason many people resist, delay, or refuse to consider it without knowing what they are missing.

Thankfully, that was not the case with the Zimbles. Mickey immediately said he thought having hospice care at home "sounds like a good idea." Sandy was initially reluctant "to have strangers in my home," explaining that they were people who always took care of things themselves. She was more than happy to care for Mickey. As I listened quietly to Sandy explain her concerns, she got around to admitting that, despite her sense of privacy, she knew that she would need help.

I only had to suggest, "I think you should give hospice a try," for her to agree.

It took a lot more encouragement on my part—bordering on stern insistence—for Sandy to agree to contact their four adult children and, if they offered, to allow them to help care for Mickey during their father's first weeks at home from the hospital.

She reluctantly acquiesced and called her children that afternoon. She was soon glad she had taken my advice. Their son and one of their three daughters arrived the very next day. Their presence immediately lightened the physical and emotional weight of Mickey's illness and care.

As soon as the C. Diff infection cleared, we stopped the metronidazole and started Mickey on prednisone to decrease inflammation around the tumors in his liver. His pain decreased and appetite reawakened. He developed a new love of chocolate-covered raisins, which he credited with giving him energy and raising his red blood cell count. He also developed a near obsession with Sudoku, through which he whiled away the hours and days waiting for his strength to return. Our team remained in close touch with the hospice medical director and the Zimbles' primary hospice nurse. As Mickey's symptoms diminished, we collaborated by phone with the hospice team on adjustments to his medications. Through late June and July, Mickey gained weight and energy, and finally set down his Sudoku books in favor of taking walks and even golfing a few rounds. In early August he was well enough to officially "graduate" from hospice.

On the day in mid-August that Mickey returned to see Dr. Ernstoff at the Norris Cotton Cancer Center, I also saw him in clinic. Mickey's face was round and slightly puffy, his hair a bit sparse, and his skin almost translucent—all side effects of the prednisone, which was making him feel so good. He said that he had had "the best summer in memory." He knew that he couldn't stay on this dose of prednisone much longer because of the swelling, high blood pressure, and insulin-resistance (diabetagenic) side effects. He was eager to have more treatment for the tumors in his liver and hoping that Dr. Ernstoff still had "something up his sleeve."

In fact, he did. By October, after three cycles of docetaxel, a potent anticancer drug, the tumors in his liver seemed to melt away. We began tapering his prednisone dose, and he and Sandy began making plans to winter at their home in Florida.

When Reed Abelson called Sandy in February 2007, Mickey was out playing golf. Reed tried again two days later with the same result. "He's out there walking and playing nine holes of golf," Sandy told Reed. And so that was what she wrote. The title of her article that ran in the *New York Times* on February 10, 2007, was "There Is Life After Hospice, and Even Golf in Florida for Some."

What happened to Mickey is not all that uncommon. Research now shows that many people live longer with hospice care. A research team led by Dr. Stephen Connor analyzed Medicare data from 1998 through 2002 for patients who had a serious diagnosis, such as congestive heart failure and cancer, three years or more before their death. Dr. Connor's team then compared the survival of those who received hospice care to those with the same conditions who did not. Overall, patients receiving hospice care lived an average of twenty-nine days longer. The survival advantage was statistically significant for people with congestive heart failure (who lived an average of eighty-one days longer), lung cancer (thirty-nine days longer), and pancreatic cancer (twenty-one days longer) with positive survival trends for those with colon, breast, and prostate cancer. Perhaps equally important, hospice care was not associated with shorter length of life for any group of patients.

A growing body of clinical research suggests that for people with advanced illness, improvements in quality of life go hand in hand with extending the length of life.

At Dartmouth, a palliative care research team led by Dr. Marie Bakitas, whose doctorate is in nursing science, enrolled 322 patients with advanced cancer receiving standard oncology care. Patients gave permission to be assigned by chance to one of two groups. One group received phone-based visits with a nurse who inquired about their symptoms and provided education, coordination of care, and supportive counseling for living with their illness. The other group did not. The main focus of the study was to assess the effects of this simple, less comprehensive, and relatively inexpensive palliative intervention on people's well-being and health care use. On average, people receiving this "low-dose" palliative intervention had significantly higher mood and self-reported quality of life, while there was no significant effect on symptom intensity (which was low in both groups) or on total health services used through the end of life. The study was not designed to investigate the impact on survival, yet it found that median length of life was 14 months in the intervention group and 8.5 months for those receiving standard oncology care. By the study's completion at three years, similar numbers of patients in both groups had died.

Convincing evidence of the capacity of palliative care to simultaneously improve quality and extend length of life came from a study by oncologist Dr. Jennifer Temel and associates at Massachusetts General

Hospital. After giving their permission to participate in the study, 151 patients who had been recently diagnosed with incurable metastatic lung cancer were randomly assigned to receive cancer treatment with or without concurrent palliative care. This was team-based, "full-dose" palliative care of the sort that our team at Dartmouth provides. Patients receiving palliative care experienced substantially lower incidence of depression and higher quality of life on three standardized, multidimensional questionnaires. The most striking finding was that patients in the palliative care group lived a median of 11.6 months, compared to 8.9 months in the usual care group. A 2.7-month survival advantage might not seem dramatic, but this magnitude of therapeutic effect would be considered a major advance if it were attributable to a new chemotherapy treatment for people with late stages of lung, pancreas, breast, or colon cancer. In Dr. Temel's study, patients in the intervention group were less likely to receive aggressive cancer treatments within two weeks of their death and more likely to receive hospice care at home.

This study rightly made headlines when it was published and generated substantial discussion. It now seemed possible that team-based palliative care extended life to a degree comparable to newer immune-based chemotherapy drugs that may cost $6,000 to $10,000 per month and can cause rashes, bleeding, infection, and other life-threatening side effects. In contrast, team-based palliative care for a patient and family typically costs several hundred dollars per month and does not cause rashes, bleeding, or infections. With palliative care, quantity and quality of life are not at odds; indeed, being comfortable is considered a key to living longer.

Mickey's good quality of life continued into early spring. Dr. Ernstoff spoke with a specialist in neuroendocrine tumors in Florida and together they arranged for Mickey to continue receiving chemotherapy infusions every three weeks during the winter and spring in Florida. During the last days of March he felt weaker and his appetite was poor. His oncologist in Florida repeated blood tests and a CT scan, and told

Mickey and Sandy that the tests now showed that the cancer was progressing despite the chemotherapy. He said that it was now time again to bring in hospice care.

This time, almost magically, to Sandy's surprise and relief, all four of their children arrived at their Florida home that same night. They explained to their parents that they were staying for the duration. The duration turned out to be just a handful of days. His hospice nurse visited in the morning to review plans for managing his symptoms and to make certain that everything they needed was in place. On Friday, April 6, 2007, Mickey said he didn't have the energy to get up and get dressed.

In the early afternoon he became restless and uncomfortable, and insisted he needed to get out of bed. He confided to his son, Barry, that he was dying. Barry assured him that everything was in place and that he and his sisters were all there to help care for him and to support their mom and one another. The hospice nurse returned at 3:30 in the afternoon. She placed a few drops of highly concentrated oral morphine under his tongue and gave him a small dose of lorazepam solution. He was more comfortable within minutes.

Mickey died peacefully at 5:22 p.m. with Sandy and their children sitting around his bed.

Over lunch with Sandy, nearly three years later, I asked her to reflect on their experience. Sandy said she still gets sad whenever she thinks of his dying but feels Mickey's last months were a gift. "Through palliative care he did have wonderful quality of life. When you met him in the hospital, he never dreamt that he would go to Florida again. He never dreamt he would walk or play golf!"

When I asked Sandy what she thought had been helpful to Mickey's care, she was emphatic that the quality of life and length of his life were connected. By relieving his pain, decreasing the swelling in his legs so that he could walk, and adjusting his medications so that his appetite came back, she felt he'd regained his will to live.

Were there lessons she would tell others? I asked. She was also

emphatic. "If you hadn't made me involve my children and my family—
I wouldn't have done it, because I was 'the mother.' I'd say, 'Oh, my kids
are busy.'" (At the time, their "kids" were all in their fifties.) "But you
said, 'They have to be here.' So, I listened to you."

She has become a true believer.

"Now I say the same thing to all my friends who have someone who
is ill. It is important that people know that they cannot be modest. They
have to have the support of family to rally around and work it out. That
is something that you taught me, Ira. I have included my kids in everything since, but it was something I never did before because I was the
mother."

When any one person becomes sick, a family inevitably experiences
the illness. Each and every member of a person's emotional family feels
an impact in his or her own way. I often say to families, "You are each
going to experience this as individuals. You might as well go through it
together."

Although the evidence continues to build, it is still surprising to
many people that hospice and palliative care help patients live longer.
Hospice, particularly, is associated in people's minds with dying. That
is a result of Medicare's regulatory restrictions, but hospice is—and
should be—much more. Because it is funded by Medicare—under specific eligibility criteria—hospice programs are widespread and the most
highly developed and available way of delivering palliative care in the
United States.

In many areas, hospice does serve patients in hospitals and nursing
homes. However, for the most part in the United States, hospice cares
for patients who wish to stay at home through the end of life. It is often
said that the main problem with hospice care is that you have to be
dying to get it.

Hospital-based palliative care programs are much newer. A few
years earlier the sort of care that our palliative care team provided to
Mickey and Sandy Zimble would not have been available. Without the

fairly intensive level of care that our team provided while he was in the hospital—we saw him at least daily and sometimes two or more times when he was in pain or anxious—Mickey might well have died within a week or two of going home.

With little public awareness or fanfare, in recent years, hospital-based palliative care programs have flourished. Almost all hospitals of two hundred beds or more—and many smaller hospitals—now have at least a small palliative care program.

Clinical outcome studies suggest that palliative care can alleviate pain, shortness of breath, and other distressing symptoms among seriously ill people, enhance their quality of life, and improve satisfaction on the part of patients and families.

Key components of palliative care, such as family meetings to clarify goals of care, clear communication about prognosis and expected outcomes, and counseling related to life completion and closure can decrease conflict over treatment decisions. These elements of care have been shown to diminish post-traumatic stress among family members after a patient has been in the ICU, and may lighten the weight of grief family members experience after a patient dies.

In another study, Dr. Bakitas's research team at Dartmouth-Hitchcock Medical Center reviewed charts of one hundred patients who died in our hospital during 2008. Thirty-two patients had been seen at least once by our clinical palliative care team. The patients served by our palliative care team were more likely to have an advance directive document on file (72 percent vs. 48 percent) and less likely to die in an ICU (25 percent vs. 67 percent). They averaged fewer invasive interventions, such as CPR, intubation and assisted ventilation, kidney dialysis, chemotherapy, and medically administered nutrition, but were significantly more likely to have been visited by a social worker or chaplain. Importantly, families of patients who were served by our palliative care team were more likely to be present at the time of death.

When we first meet patients, we often cannot predict the course of their illness. Even when cure is out of reach, for some people, like Mickey Zimble, late-stage treatments can help stem the tide of disease or enable people to maintain an even keel. Part of our role becomes helping people stay the course of treatment, managing practical problems, and alleviating any side effects and complications that arise.

I often meet people who know full well that they are dying but want to stay alive for a special event. Paul Gilliam fit that description. In his early fifties, Paul was being slowly killed by colon cancer that had blocked his bowel and caused puddles of infected fluid to form in his pelvis. He was miserable, and desperate to stay alive to attend his only daughter's wedding. Our palliative plan of care included daily IV antibiotics and monthly CT scans so that the interventional radiologists could reposition catheters that drained his infections. To control pain he wore a fanny pack with a small portable pump that delivered a continuous IV infusion of hydromorphone and had a PCA button that he could push to give himself an extra dose up to every ten minutes, when he needed it. Because he was younger than sixty-five and had insurance through his employer, he was not bound by Medicare's "either-or" restrictions for hospice care. Therefore, Paul was admitted to hospice and the hospice team in his community coordinated his health care at home, including making sure that his antibiotics and hydromorphone were administered as prescribed. His insurance paid for his scans, procedures, and hospital bills separately.

All of these measures enabled Paul to live with his cancer and keep his infections at bay. Still, he remained discouraged that he could not receive more chemotherapy. To him chemotherapy represented hope for living longer. However, Paul's oncologist had been clear that because of his infections, any further compromise of his immune system would be deadly.

There was another perspective that I wanted to offer. "Paul, for what it is worth, when people have been fighting cancer for a long time, as you have, there often comes a point at which they may live longer if they decide to live *with their cancer* rather than continue to fight *against their cancer*. What I mean is that if a person is tired and run-down, more chemotherapy may not be in his or her best interests and may actually shorten the person's life.

"Oncologists tend to start with the most effective chemotherapy they have for a patient's cancer. Second-, third-, and fourth-line treatments may be less effective or carry more side effects. When cancer grows despite chemotherapy or when it recurs, the situation may become one of diminishing returns on a person's investment of limited time and energy. Since most chemotherapy affects normal cells as well as cancer cells, these medications can take a toll on one's general health—something I know you know all too well."

"I know this in my head, Dr. Byock," Paul said, "but when I get home, on the days I feel better, it drives me crazy that I am not doing something to try to live longer."

These are feelings I commonly hear people express.

"I hear you, Paul," I replied, "but please consider that what you need most—certainly right now, and possibly in the weeks ahead—is to concentrate on getting the best nutrition you can, and both rest and exercise when you are able. People are more than their organ systems. Being comfortable and emotionally well within yourself is also important to your general health and to living longer. I believe that is why studies have shown that people who receive hospice care actually tend to live longer than people who don't."

In Paul's situation it worked. With intensive supportive care he lived to attend and enjoy his daughter's wedding and a few months more.

When I approached Alonzo Scarza about hospice care, I knew it would be a sensitive conversation. At seventy-two years of age, Alonzo had never slowed down. Now he had been diagnosed with esophageal cancer that had spread throughout the lining of his stomach. The surgeon who had tried—and failed—to remove the tumor told him that his stomach resembled a deflated leather football and was every bit as stiff.

Alonzo couldn't eat. The surgeon had placed a feeding tube, which traversed his abdominal wall and could deliver nutrient solution directly into his jejunum. But Alonzo's gut would not tolerate more than 300 or 400 calories a day, nowhere near enough to keep him alive in the long run.

When I first met him, seven months earlier, Alonzo was still stocky and built like a football player. I wasn't surprised when he told me that he'd been a star defensive lineman in high school. There were half a dozen photos of Alonzo taped to his hospital room wall, usually grinning, with his arm around one of his kids or wife or sister. Except for a midlife belly, he had retained his muscular frame through his adult years. Now, like his shriveled stomach, he appeared deflated. His usually smooth dark skin had a ruddy purplish hue and cobbled texture of a rash caused by one of the chemotherapy medications. It took a conscious effort for him to turn himself in bed and he needed help transferring to the commode or recliner in his hospital room.

Our team had met Alonzo during previous hospitalizations. He was almost always animated. Alonzo was proudly Italian-American, but he frequently reminded me of Anthony Quinn in the film *Zorba the Greek*. Loud, exuberant, arms open. This was his third time in the hospital in the past two months and his fifth time since February. This time it was for a "port infection." The reusable injection site implanted under his skin for administering chemotherapy and other medications had become colonized with MRSA, a *Staphylococcus aureus* bacteria that is resistant to nearly all antibiotics. Having MRSA bacteria in his bloodstream was acutely life-threatening. But in Alonzo's case, the MRSA infection was already under control and on the way to being cured. Treating it had required removing the port and long intravenous catheter to which it was connected, and two weeks of antibiotics through new IVs in his forearms or wrists that were replaced every few days. Things had gone well and he was due to be discharged in just a couple of days. I expected him to be upbeat and talkative, but his mood was unusually dark. Alonzo was frustrated, he said, because Dr. King, his primary oncologist, had stopped by his hospital room and explained, yet again, that he could not have more chemotherapy.

He had been diagnosed with cancer in early fall, little more than half a year ago, but said, "It seems like another lifetime," adding with his arm raised for emphasis, "before the worst fucking winter of my life."

When he was diagnosed, even though his cancer appeared to be confined to the juncture of his esophagus and stomach, the odds were long against his cancer being cured. Still, aggressive treatments seemed worth a try. During the discussion at Gastro-Intestinal Tumor Board, the hope was that chemotherapy might shrink the tumor enough for an oncologic surgeon to take out his lower esophagus and most of his stomach and fashion a small pouch to function as a neo-stomach. If all went well, he would be able to eat nearly normally (small frequent meals) within six months to a year. Unfortunately, instead of things going well, his first round of chemotherapy was a nightmare. He had terrible mucositis—the lining of his mouth and throat became inflamed and then raw, as if they had been burned and the skin sloughed off—and the chemotherapy caused his blood counts to plummet. After eleven days in the hospital he had recovered enough to go home. A week later he was readmitted with swollen legs, readily diagnosed by ultrasound as clots in the veins of both his legs and his pelvis. Adding insult to injury, an allergic reaction to heparin, the medication he was given to dissolve the clots and prevent new ones, caused his platelet counts to fall even further than they had from the recent chemotherapy. This put him at high risk of bleeding. Thankfully, a different blood-thinning medication worked well. His platelet count rose and, once again, he was well enough to go home.

Two weeks later, he restarted chemotherapy. At least twice a month, one of the nurse practitioners from our team, Betty Priest or Helen Walek, had an appointment with Alonzo on a day he came for cancer treatments. At least twice during the past four months, they had gently raised the topic of hospice care with Mr. Scarza. But to Alonzo, hospice meant giving up. He was having no part of it.

Alonzo was a self-described stubborn man—"I'm hardheaded, no sense denying it," he said—but he was hard not to like. He was a quintessential character, a second-generation Italian-American whose facial expressions, bighearted smile, way with words, and life story were positively cinematic. His father was just six years old when he came to America, through Ellis Island, with Alonzo's grandparents. Alonzo was the same age when he, his father, Anthony, and his mother and younger sister were interred during World War II.

After the war, his family moved to Reno, Nevada, and his father worked in construction, becoming a foreman for a thriving building company. Alonzo followed in his dad's footsteps and learned to run heavy machinery. He, too, became a foreman and then supervisor of major construction projects. Finally, he started his own company. He loved his work and his employees—and they loved him. He succeeded in business and, it seemed, in life. Besides his work, Alonzo loved horses. Mostly he loved owning racehorses and betting on them; the latter passion he retained through his illness.

In the hospital, on days he felt reasonably well, he was a fount of captivating stories about the horses he had loved and races his horses and jockeys had won or lost. One knew when he felt poorly, because he wouldn't regale you with stories. Even on his worst days, Alonzo was patient and uncomplaining.

He married for the first time in his late thirties, and he and his wife had a son whom they named after his deceased father. Tragically, his wife and son were killed in a car accident when little Anthony was just nine. Alonzo grieved, but went on. In telling me about that time in his life, he said he knew that life was not fair and he did not expect only joy. He remained single for nearly two decades, absorbed in his business and "the ponies," until 1992, when he met and fell in love with Carla. The daughter of a close friend, Carla was twenty-two years younger than Alonzo. They married and soon Carla gave birth to a little girl, Toni, who was now eight years old and the apple of Alonzo's eye.

During the fall and winter from hell when he was hospitalized, first for his surgery, then for the side effects of chemotherapy, and clotting and low platelet counts—whenever things did not look good, Alonzo would explain that he was fighting to stay around "for Carla and Toni." Whenever one of us, or Dr. King, asked him what his goals were, his answer was "to get stronger" so that he could have more treatments.

On this day, however, it was time to bring up hospice again. We had finished our routine of discussing his abdominal and mid-back pain, whether he had significant relief when he pushed the PCA "pain button," and, on average, whether he'd been using it any less since we had adjusted the continuous dose yesterday. Yes, he was using it considerably less. We asked how he'd slept (not so well, due to being awakened whenever his IV pump beeped and at five a.m. to have his blood pressure checked) and whether he had gotten out of the room at all yesterday (yes, for a few laps around the ward and one walk to get a *Boston Globe* at the store on the medical center's Main Street).

Alonzo knew that he was getting ready for discharge, but he was not eager for it. He felt secure in the hospital. The nurses knew him well and universally liked him—and they were always just a push of his call button away.

There was no good medical reason for him to stay in the hospital. The MRSA had been defeated, the causes of his various symptoms and general decline were known, and symptomatic treatments were in place. No further tests or scans were planned. Likewise, there were no plans at present to treat his cancer. He was far too weak to receive more chemotherapy. Dr. King had been explicit that he would need to gain at least fifteen pounds and be able to walk without assistance—except with the aid of a walker—before he would consider giving him another dose of chemo. This was a bone of contention for Alonzo.

I knew I had my work cut out for me.

"Alonzo, I have to have another serious conversation with you about going home."

He looked at me and nodded imperceptibly.

"Your infection has cleared up. Your pain is pretty well controlled." I spoke slowly. Although I had other patients to see, this discussion could not be rushed. In the practice of palliative care this conversation was a medical intervention every bit as important as an operation is to a surgeon.

"In sending you home, I want to make sure you are getting the best care possible. At this time, I believe that includes hospice care. I know that's a sensitive topic," I said, "but I want you to hear me out."

Those last words had not left my mouth before he gave me a look that he'd give a guy who was trying to sell him a lame horse.

"I don't know how many times I have to tell you, I am not giving up. I will walk back into that office—mark my words," he said.

"Alonzo, you are a strong man. I *have* been listening. We all have. We are all on board with helping you get there. We think it is a long shot, but you have a lot to live for and you have beaten long odds in your life before.

"It will take a lot for you to get stronger. You need help with your nutrition and medications and with getting around. Look at all the care that the nurses have been doing for you here. When you go home, you are going to continue to need your pain and nausea medications, and the blood thinner injections, and the J-tube [jejunostomy tube] infusion. Carla is good with all of this, but it's a lot for one person to do. I want her to have all the help she can get."

I explained that hospice is the highest level of home care there is for people in his situation. "It's like home health care on steroids," I said. "I know that you don't want to hear about it because hospice is intended for people who are dying, but there's a loophole." I paused. He looked up. Now I had his attention.

"Officially, you do not need to die to get hospice care; you just have to be sick enough so that no one would be surprised if, six months from now, you had died. Here's the deal. On the papers that they will give you to sign, it will say that to qualify for hospice you must acknowledge that you have a condition that is likely to take your life 'if the disease runs its natural course.'" I made air quotes with two fingers of each hand as I spoke. "The words 'if the disease runs its natural course' on the admission form comes right from the law that made Medicare start paying for hospice care.

"What you have been trying to do—what we have all been trying to do—is to change the natural course of this disease. That is still the goal. But let's look at the trends, Alonzo. Months ago you were visiting the stables and track every day, but during the past six months your strength and appetite and weight have gradually declined." Now I traced a set of stairs in the air with my index finger, each step headed down.

"Let's face it. If we are unable to change the natural course of the disease, no one will be surprised if you will have died six months from now. Isn't that right?"

Our eyes met. He hesitated only a second. "Yes. That's right." He nodded.

"I just don't want too many people in our home. I think we can get by with the nurse coming a couple of times a week." This was a second level of resistance and might mean I was making progress.

"I want to answer that in a few ways. First, it is lousy to have your privacy invaded. All I can say is that we will ask the hospice team to keep things to a minimum and respect your privacy and your family's privacy. In my experience, once people actually meet the hospice nurse who will help care for them, he or she stops being an idea and becomes a person. Familiarity builds quickly, and before long it doesn't feel like an intrusion to have the nurse visit.

"I also want you to know that I am bringing this up because I *have been* listening. Even with hospice involved, you will have more privacy at home than in here. My worry is that if we send you home with routine home health care—a nurse to visit once or twice a week, it will not be enough support and there will be a time when we'll be rushing to catch up to your and Carla's needs. If something happens—maybe a bad episode of pain or your IV becoming unplugged—you could very likely end up back in the hospital. When situations like that occur, Alonzo, the truth is sometimes people conclude that 'we can't manage at home'"—my air quotes were back—"and the person who is ill ends up in a nursing home. I don't want that to happen here."

I realized that I was scaring him, but I have seen situations similar to his play out in this fashion far too many times not to warn him about what might lie ahead.

I explained that hospice care just might help him live longer—that ironic as it might seem, hospice would give him the best chance of meeting his goal of getting strong enough to receive more chemotherapy. I was honest that even with hospice, I thought the chances were small. Still, I was doing my best to get him to let the hospice team in the door.

"The hospice program can send a nurse in two or three times a week if all is well, but more frequently if needed. A physical therapist from hospice can see what sort of equipment might help you transfer out of bed. They can adjust your J-tube infusion so that as your body tolerates it, you can hopefully gain some weight. If all goes well and you gain the weight and get stronger, you can simply 'graduate from hospice' and get more chemotherapy. There is nothing wrong with that. If you do not get stronger, you will already know the team that can best support you and Carla and Toni through the end of your life.

"Capishe?" I asked in my best Jersey Italian.

"Yeah, I understand," he replied, nodding his head as he continued to ponder the change in his situation. His mouth was in a tight smile, but he did not look happy; rather, he looked resolved, as if his horse had just crossed the line fourth. "It is what it is, eh, Doc?"

Few people in Alonzo's situation do graduate from hospice. It may be as few as one in twenty. Mickey Zimble was one of the lucky ones. Most people in Alonzo's predicament go on to die at home, with hospice care continuing. Alonzo did, only three weeks after being discharged. He was at home, comfortable, and from his family's report, at peace.

My favorite example of someone being referred to palliative care, including hospice, and living longer is not Paul Gilliam or Mickey Zimble or Art Buchwald; it is my cousin, Edith Glikin.

Norman Glikin, Edith's late husband, was my mother's cousin. Edith and Norman were my parents' best friends. Growing up, they and their children, Sandy and Susie, were my favorite relatives. Our families spent a lot of time together. As a young boy, during a summer week I spent at their home playing with Sandy, Edith taught me to ride a bicycle, for which I am eternally grateful.

In late January 2004, at the age of eighty-three, Edith underwent heart surgery. Things went well during surgery, but she had a very difficult recovery, marked by prolonged heart failure, breathing difficulties, dangerous cardiac arrhythmias, and profound depression. She was in the hospital for weeks, much of the time in pain and generally miserable. During the first weeks, she had to have a thoracentesis performed on three occasions to remove fluid around her lungs. In the larger scheme of medical procedures, it is not a big deal. But it was to Edith. In an X-ray suite, sitting on a cold table, her robe was removed and the sides of her chest were swabbed with iodine solution (also cold) as a disinfectant. A small shot of local anesthetic was injected in a dime-size area at a site on her mid-back, underneath which lay a pool of fluid. The radiologist passed a long, wide needle (roughly twice the diameter of a spaghetti noodle) between her ribs until fluid was returned. Then a guide wire was passed through the needle, the needle was withdrawn, and a firm, tapered plastic catheter about the gauge of macaroni was threaded over the guide wire and into the pleural effusion that had collected between the linings of the chest wall and lungs. The guide wire was then withdrawn and the outer end of the catheter was connected to

a stopcock. Being very careful to maintain negative pressure on the catheter at all times, the physician who performed the procedure withdrew
fluid into a large syringe. When he had drained all he could, the catheter
and syringe were removed and a watertight dressing was applied to her
skin. Then he repeated the procedure on the other side.

Edith lost all her appetite while in the hospital and, therefore,
wasn't getting the calories or protein she needed to get stronger. She
was unable—or refused—to participate in physical therapy. Edith
thought she was dying and repeatedly asked her children—Sandy and
Susan and their spouses—to let her go home. Several of her immediate family members, including Sandy, who is a pediatrician, his wife,
Jenny, and sister, Susan, who are both nurses, worried that she might be
dying. Edith's cardiologist disagreed. He explained that she merely had
a shocked heart syndrome. It was unfortunate, he said, but it happens
sometimes. While bothersome, he was sure she would eventually get
better. With this assurance, the family acquiesced and prevailed upon
Edith to go to a rehabilitation center. The first one was awful and was
too far from her daughter, Susan, so after a few weeks she was transferred to another.

Things went from bad to worse and Edith, clearly failing to thrive,
was readmitted to the hospital. Now there was concern that she needed
a PEG tube to supplement her nutrition. Antidepressants that had been
prescribed during her first hospitalization were changed. Edith continued to decline.

I had been staying in touch with the family by phone but had not
been part of decision-making conversations. By early March 2004,
Jenny Glikin called me and asked me to weigh in. She described Edith
as deteriorating in body and spirit. Her heart failure was stable, but she
was not eating, exceedingly weak due to her surgery and decondition-
ing, and getting weaker.

I asked Jenny whether she would be surprised if Edith died within
the next six months.

"Not at all. I would be surprised if she were alive in six months!" Jenny replied.

This is a slight variation of what's come to be known as "the surprise question"—"Would you be surprised if this patient died in the next year?"—that has been promulgated by palliative care physician Joanne Lynn as a simple way of screening for eligibility for palliative care. Studies have shown that a physician's response to the surprise question is a significant prognostic indicator—that is, a predictor of a person's life expectancy—in cancer and kidney failure, as well as in a large primary care practice.

I suggested that we consider referring Edith to hospice and Jenny thought it made good sense. Her general debility combined with her heart failure would make her eligible under Medicare. When Sandy and Jenny approached Edith's cardiologist, he told them the idea was unheard of. When I subsequently called him, he initially said the same thing to me. However, when I asked him the "surprise question," he had to admit that he wouldn't be shocked if she died in the next six months, or even the next three months. He agreed that she had been declining. Her performance status was awful, her serum albumin was less than 2—an objective sign of malnourishment. I explained that the family was willing to care for her around the clock (including hiring nurses' aides to sit with her at night) and that the hospice program would send skilled nurses to weigh her and take her blood pressure and pulse, examine her with special attention to her breathing and edema, and help manage her medications, including her furosemide (Lasix) and potassium. A physical therapist with hospice would see her twice a week and would teach both Edith and her family strengthening exercises. This time, he reluctantly agreed—or acquiesced.

It all worked. Once at home, Edith's mood improved. She started eating. She worked with the physical therapist and her nurses' aides and did her exercises faithfully. Her improvement was slow but steady. Her shocked heart syndrome gradually resolved. Her swelling subsided and her depression lifted. Within three weeks she was up and around with a walker; within five weeks, she was feeling better than she had been before surgery. She graduated from hospice.

Fourteen months after her surgery, I danced with Edith at a family wedding. For me, Edith's experience epitomizes the connection between higher quality of life and survival. Like Mickey Zimble, she recovered her will to live and, thereafter, she recovered. We recently celebrated Edith's ninetieth birthday. She has just had the battery of her implanted cardiac defibrillator replaced. While she was in the hospital I interviewed her about her thoughts on having been a hospice patient.

She said her cardiologist, whom she sees every six months and likes very much, still thinks I am crazy. She laughed out loud when she told me that he teases her every time she comes in for her routine appointments. "He's clueless! I wouldn't be here if it wasn't for you and hospice!" she joyfully exclaimed. Her children and I would make the same decision again.

5.

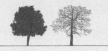

Morbidity and Mortality

Today's case involves a twenty-seven-year-old man with newly diagnosed HIV-AIDS who presented with progressive bilateral pneumonia that progressed to fulminate ARDS [acute respiratory distress syndrome]. The case involved complex medical complications and decision-making and entailed considerable suffering."

Dr. Antonia Altomare stood behind the podium, looking up at her audience in a large lecture hall at Dartmouth-Hitchcock Medical Center. The auditorium was an academic amphitheater and the event was the time-honored tradition of the monthly Morbidity and Mortality conference.

In the culture of medicine, Morbidity and Mortality conferences occupy a privileged position. M&M conferences (or just M&Ms in the vernacular of medicine) are the places where bad outcomes, usually potentially avoidable serious complications or deaths, and even frank mistakes are openly discussed for the sake of improving practice and quality of care. In recognition of their time-honored value as quality improvement and continuing education activities, many states' laws grant M&M conferences special protection from being discoverable in civil malpractice litigation. These are weighty events. Not surprisingly, the prospect of presenting a case for discussion at an M&M conference can be terrifying for physicians-in-training.

The tradition began in the field of surgery where the warrior culture is particularly strong. To this day departments of surgery in most teaching hospitals require all staff surgeons and surgical residents to attend the regularly scheduled monthly M&M conferences. And, consistent with surgical culture, surgery M&Ms are regularly scheduled for six thirty on a weekday morning. At that early hour, before an auditorium of one's surgical mentors and peers, the armor of invincibility and infallibility is dropped or simply disappears. Cases are presented by a physician representing the patient's treating team, and questions and comments are solicited from the surgeons in attendance. The focus is tightly on the quality of care provided. Criticisms are plain spoken and not personal—in fact, the process is deliberately nonpersonal—but questions and comments can cut deeply, something surgeons do best.

Many departments of internal medicine have adopted the practice with minor modifications. Internal Medicine M&Ms tend to occur during daylight hours and criticisms tend to be less blunt. However, presenting a case at M&M is still not for the faint of heart.

One of the pleasures of practicing where I do is the opportunity to interact with bright, energetic, deeply committed physicians-in-training. I enjoy teaching and practicing with them—and learning from them. Dr. Altomare is among the very brightest residents I have ever encountered. Hardworking, smart, and serious, Antonia is a petite, dark-haired young woman, who, in addition to her intellect and thoughtful, meticulous work, is known for being consistently cheerful, somehow even during brutally long days and nights at the hospital.

This Internal Medicine M&M conference offered Antonia a high-profile opportunity to teach her fellow residents and her faculty alike. After residency, Antonia was going on to fellowship training in infectious disease and had chosen this case partly because of the many infectious problems that the patient had experienced. But there was more to it than that. Antonia had e-mailed me two weeks before the conference to let me know she was going to present Daren's case. Being familiar with the patient and his family, I thought it was a courageous choice. Few cases are as wrenching as Daren's. In saying clearly that it "entailed considerable suffering," Antonia had crafted a gutsy opening in a most challenging academic venue.

She continued, "Daren McCallum, the pseudonym I'll use in referring to our patient, presented to the hospital on April 23 last year. He had been seen at an urgent care center in Minneapolis, where he lives, for complaints of a nonproductive cough, rhinorrhea, and fever twice in the month prior to admission. Treatment with oral azithromycin resolved the fever and improved his symptoms for several days. However, within a week his symptoms recurred. Eleven days prior to admission, he saw an internist in Minneapolis. A chest X-ray showed bilateral infiltrates and he was treated with moxifloxacin and prednisone, and improved only slightly. During the week, he flew to Vermont to stay with his parents. His cough worsened, low-grade fevers recurred, and he developed shortness of breath. On the morning of admission, he saw his family's primary care physician who was concerned about the worsening of his respiratory status. A chest X-ray now showed more dense infiltrates bilaterally. His doctor arranged for an urgent consultation with the Infectious Disease clinic here. The patient was admitted from the ID clinic."

As she spoke, PowerPoint slides with bulleted highlights of the sequence of events appeared on a large screen behind her left shoulder; his symptoms, dates of his visits, lab and X-ray tests, and medications prescribed. Each slide was replete with medical terms, abbreviations, and jargon that would have been undecipherable to nonclinicians. Even for the majority of the physician audience who do not practice infectious disease, several abbreviations and medications were unfamiliar. This only heightened our interest. In the 1980s and early 1990s patients with HIV disease and life-threatening opportunistic infections were common. However, in the United States and many of the developed countries, since the advent of highly active antiretroviral therapy, or HAART, in 1996, the incidence of full-blown AIDS has fallen sharply. For a majority of Americans who are HIV positive—HIV+ for short— the infection has become a manageable, chronic condition. And for many HIV+ people who are taking HAART medications, the infection causes no apparent health problems. Indeed, Daren was one of only a handful of patients with HIV-related conditions that our Palliative Care Service team has helped care for in the past few years.

Antonia presented the clinical story as it had unfolded to the physicians who had admitted Daren to the hospital slightly more than seven months earlier. She summarized his admission H&P (med-speak for the history and physical examination), which included basic information about his past history, including medically pertinent details of his personal and social life, all of which she related in a matter-of-fact manner. We learned that Daren lived in the Twin Cities area, and worked as a buyer for an electronics firm. He was single, sexually active with men, a nonsmoker, who occasionally drank one or two beers in the evening, and had never used illicit drugs. He had not traveled outside the country in the past three years, had no pets, no close exposure to birds, and no history of exposure to asbestos or other respiratory toxins.

The physical examination note that she read described Daren on the day of his hospital admission as appearing acutely ill. Even with 2 liters per minute of pure oxygen blowing through cannulae in his nostrils, he was slightly short of breath with exertion. He could speak in full sentences, but they tended to be short sentences. At times he leaned forward to brace himself with his forearms and tightened the "accessory muscles" in his neck and shoulders to help him breathe.

His past medical history was unremarkable. He had never been seriously ill and did not have asthma or a history of other respiratory problems. His only surgery and only time in the hospital was for appendicitis at age twelve. He reported being negative on a test for HIV three years ago.

For the first fifteen minutes or so Antonia presented the medical details of the case, which were fascinating to those of us whose practices involve taking care of seriously ill people. (If there was ever a time and place in which morbid fascination was entirely appropriate, this was certainly it.)

She showed a grid of his laboratory tests and initial X-rays. His white blood cell count was modestly elevated at 12,700, abnormal but not alarming. His chest X-ray was more impressive, showing patches of white infiltrates scattered throughout his right and left lungs. However, the X-ray images were nonspecific. A large number of viruses or bacteria or inflammatory conditions can cause this pattern. Knowing that his most recent HIV test was positive helped narrow the diagnosis, but the number of germs to which HIV+ patients are at risk for is still long—and worrisome.

During the first hours of his hospitalization, multiple laboratory tests were sent—blood cultures for bacteria and fungi, and antibody tests for common viruses. A CD4 count (an index of the T lymphocytes affected by the virus) and viral load assay were sent to better define the extent of his HIV disease. He was started on IV antibiotics for presumed Pneumocystis carinii pneumonia (or PCP) infection, a frequent consequence of AIDS that causes significant inflammation in the lungs of affected people. For that reason he was also restarted on prednisone, an anti-inflammatory steroid medicine.

Early in Daren's care the question of when to begin antiretroviral treatments against HIV was raised. Antonia related a discussion among one of the infectious disease faculty physicians, a resident, Daren, and his father during which they discussed the possibility that treating the HIV virus too soon could cause inflammation and temporarily cause his lung condition to deteriorate. She presented slides with data from two published studies on IRIS, the immune reconstitution inflammatory syndrome, a paradoxical worsening of illness that can follow starting HAART drugs. The findings suggested that it is important to wait about two weeks after treating PCP or other opportunistic infections before starting highly active antiretroviral therapy. Consistent with recommendations, HAART medications were initially withheld.

Nevertheless, Daren's condition worsened. Over the next few days, despite multiple medications to fight infection and corticosteroids to quell inflammation, his oxygen requirements rose from 2 liters to 4 liters per minute. Now the tubes were drying and bothering his nose. The medical team's daily progress note on hospital day 3 includes a quote from Daren: "I can't seem to take a deep breath, I get pretty tired when I get up." The next day he got intensely short of breath simply walking from his bed to the bathroom. That day's progress note quotes Daren saying, "This is the worst experience of my life."

I inwardly winced as she read the quote. Knowing the case, I was aware his experience was about to become much worse.

By day 5 his breathing was harder and Daren appeared to be tiring out. For safety's sake, he was transferred to the intermediate care unit (ICCU), an area of the hospital where sicker patients can be watched closely through continuous cardiac and respiratory monitoring, and where nurses have only two patients to care for at any time.

Antonia projected slides containing direct quotes she had extracted from the daily notes in Daren's medical chart, written by the nurses and resident physicians who were caring for him.

"Patient commented that he feels like he is probably still in shock with receiving the news about HIV. His father as well states it will take time to absorb it all. He feels that the immediate focus is getting Daren well. After that he will focus on how his son's life may be impacted."

"Patient is wondering what life will be like for him once he is out of the hospital and well. Patient does not know anyone who has HIV."

"Daren still states that his spirits are good but recognizes that he is probably still overwhelmed with the events of the past week."

In the afternoon of Daren's tenth day in the hospital, he had a fit of coughing—not unusual during this time—but suddenly became severely short of breath. The HERT team was called and responded within four minutes. On physical exam Daren had subcutaneous crepitus in his neck and underarms—meaning that his skin was puffy and, when touched, felt crunchy, as if it were covering a layer of Rice Krispies. There were decreased breath sounds at his right chest heard through a stethoscope.

The obvious diagnosis for these physical findings was a pneumothorax or collapsed lung caused by air trapped between his lung and chest wall. That was quickly confirmed by a portable X-ray. Pneumocystis carinii pneumonia often causes blebs to form in the infected lungs. As a result, pneumothoraces are fairly common complications. Although acutely life-threatening, with prompt and proper treatment they are not terribly worrisome. With a chest tube in place and gentle negative pressure to keep the lung inflated, things usually heal as the infection resolves.

The senior resident in critical care rapidly explained to Daren what needed to be done. Daren nodded his understanding and consent. The resident swabbed Daren's right chest, injected a few milliliters of lidocaine, and made a small incision in his skin with a scalpel. Then, using broad, blunt forceps, the resident pushed between two ribs and through the muscles and outer lining of Daren's chest wall, placing a plastic chest tube into his pleural space. There was no whoosh of pressure, which told the resident and ICU nurse in the room that most of the pressure of air trapped outside his lung had dissipated into the subcutaneous fat of his thorax (hence the Rice Krispies texture).

With the chest tube in place and his respiratory status still tenuous, Daren was moved to the ICU. He was not happy about his new room. He complained about the utter lack of privacy, the constant noise, and his inability to even get out of bed to sit in a chair. However, for several days, his medical condition was relatively stable. Test results showed that

Daren had a very high HIV viral load and a very low CD4, or T-cell, count of 71 (normal is between 700 and 1,000). He had CMV or cyto-megalovirus antibodies in his blood, meaning that this nasty virus could be anywhere in his body. In patients with seriously depressed immune systems, including people with HIV and low CD4 counts, CMV can infect, inflame, and kill tissues in the lung, liver, eye, and brain. Anti-body tests for one common opportunistic fungus, cryptococcus, was also positive, while another, toxoplasmosis, was negative. Serology assays for hepatitis B and C and for syphilis were all negative. A lumbar puncture was performed and tests showed no evidence of cryptococcus or CMV in his spinal fluid. An ophthalmologic examination showed no changes of CMV, but was concerning for HIV retinitis.

By this point, twenty-five minutes into the conference, the audience understood the medical picture and, because this was an M&M, knew that things must not have gone well. We were all keenly aware that in addition to conventional antibacterial, antifungal, and antiviral medica-tions directed at the CMV, Daren needed HAART meds to kill the HIV viruses that were killing his T-cells. Tension within the room mounted over when, in this unfolding story, the treating team had decided to start HAART. It occurred to me that the tension those of us in the audit-orium were feeling was but a faint reverberation of the stress the treat-ing team must have felt at the time. As Antonia continued to narrate the unfolding case, there was growing suspense surrounding the question, What the heck had gone wrong? We didn't have to wait long to find out.

On hospital day 15, Daren was started on Atripla, a combination of three antiretroviral medications that each acted on a separate pathway in the HIV virus's life cycle. On day 19 he had fevers and "desaturated into the low 80s," Antonia said, meaning the levels of oxygen in his blood plummeted whenever he moved. He developed another pneumothorax and needed a second chest tube to help reinflate his left lung.

On day 20, his temperature rose again, as did his need for supple-mental oxygen. He was working hard to breathe and his heart raced.

After a brief discussion among the critical care doctors, Daren, and his parents, he was sedated to unconsciousness with intravenous medications, intubated, and connected to a mechanical ventilator.

Notes in the medical chart reflected the rising sense of dread within his family.

> From an ICU nurse: "Parents are at his bedside, very shaken by the turn of events."
>
> From a social worker: "In respecting Daren's privacy and his explicit wishes, his parents have not told his older sister, who lives in Texas, that he was HIV+ or that he's in the hospital. Now they are feeling guilty for keeping her in the dark and uncertain what to do."
>
> From an ICU nurse: "They are concerned about Daren's sister who only knows that he has had pneumonia, but does not know he is hospitalized. Now that Daren is intubated, parents are concerned about resentment from their daughter for not sharing the situation. They want to respect Daren's wishes and are trying to do what he wants."
>
> From another ICU nurse later the same day: "Parents are feeling the burden of NOT having shared with anyone that Daren is hospitalized, let alone his HIV diagnosis."

Reading quotes of this nature is highly unusual for an M&M conference. Usually, there are detailed discussions involving specialized physiological, pathological, and anatomic details of cases, but deliberately devoid of emotion. I was impressed that instead of shying away from the emotional anguish of Daren's family, something that would have happened in most M&Ms, Antonia made it the focus of her presentation.

In spite of the content, the tone of her voice was businesslike and her pace deliberate. Over the next days, a raft of tests was obtained and treatments administered. Daren remained on the ventilator, sedated both for his comfort and so that he would not "buck the vent," reflexively coughing or breathing out of sync with the bellows of the machine. Very gradually his condition improved and on hospital day 25 sedation was decreased, the ventilator withdrawn, and the tube taken out of his throat. He was happy to be awake and able to talk!

And he had talking to do. His sister had learned that he was in the hospital from a Facebook posting by one of Daren's friends in Minneapolis. She immediately called their parents, who explained what had occurred. That night she was on a plane from Houston, and the next day she was at his bedside. Rather than being upset, Daren was upbeat and said he was relieved that she knew he was ill. He spoke tenderly to his family, saying he appreciated them all and nodded yes when asked if he'd consider going with them to a support group for people with HIV and their families. He did ask, however, that they keep the information about his HIV status, health, and hospitalization to their immediate family and very closest friends.

His respiratory function was still only borderline safe and he remained in the ICU under close observation, but with Daren's improvement, everyone's moods lifted. Six days later he underwent video-assisted thoracic surgery in which blebs were resected and the underlying lung sewed over. Four days later his chest tubes were removed. He was transferred to a private room, where he continued to recover.

The upswing was short-lived.

On his fifty-third day in the hospital, while flipping through a movie magazine, Daren abruptly became anxious and severely short of breath. Once again, the HERT team was called and he was rapidly sedated to unconsciousness and intubated. A chest X-ray showed that two new pneumothoraces had developed. New chest tubes were placed and repositioned, but there was little improvement. Bronchoscopy was performed, in which a flexible fiber-optic tube was snaked down his throat and into the branching windpipes in his lungs to look for mucus plugs that might be obstructing airflow. An emergency CT scan showed bilateral pulmonary emboli—clots in the major blood vessels of his lungs—and an ultrasound of his veins showed the source to be thrombotic clots that had formed in major veins of his right arm and neck.

Daren was anesthetized with high doses of pain and sedative medications. He was given a curare-like drug to paralyze his muscles so that the ventilator could optimally deliver oxygen-rich air to his swollen, increasingly stiff lungs. The pulmonary and critical care teams worked closely together. They tried several maneuvers to improve his oxygenation—nitrous oxide to decrease spasm of the pulmonary arteries and rapid cycle ventilation to move air without high pressures that could cause more blebs to burst. Nothing helped. An urgent meeting was held with Daren's family.

Notes from the social worker's chart entries reflect his parents' and sister's growing despair.

> Just prior to the meeting, Daren's father was at his bedside, expressing frustration over Daren's long, difficult medical saga. Daren's parents were both present at the meeting and they received information that they clearly were not prepared to hear. Dr. Gladstone explained that Daren's condition had worsened markedly and that he and the pulmonary team doubted he could survive.
>
> Daren had not wanted to inform anyone other than his parents of his diagnosis and only recently had he finally decided he needed to let his sister know about his illness. The extended family is unaware he is hospitalized, much less the gravity of his condition. When I spoke with his dad on Thursday it was apparent that the parents' inability to share this terrible situation with others—leaving them isolated from support—was becoming increasingly difficult for them. Parents have wanted to respect his wishes. They have been incredibly supportive and available to both Daren and his sister.

Antonia projected images of the new CT scan. Around the audience eyes widened; I heard a few soft gasps and witnessed several physicians involuntarily cringe. Now Daren's lungs had contracted away from his chest wall and consolidated into airless masses with the consistency of liver. The only air in his chest was outside his lungs or in abscesses, thin-walled pockets of infection within his lungs. Arrows had been placed on the computerized radiographs, pointing to blood clots in the pulmonary arteries.

She reviewed the immune reconstitution inflammatory syndrome, which was clearly playing a role in his spiraling downturn. The anti-retroviral medications were held for two days but, when there was no improvement, restarted. The infectious disease team reasoned that what was done was done and there was no reason not to keep killing the HIV viruses.

Antonia continued, "The next morning, hospital day 57, the Palliative Care Service was consulted."

I was the palliative care physician attending on our inpatient service that day and remember when the consult was called in. Judith Gladstone, the critical care faculty physician, asked us to meet with Daren's family to help them clarify goals of care and to support them through this difficult situation.

I could hear in her voice that this case affected her emotionally and she said so. "Our whole team is saddened. We thought he was going to pull through and do well. It is disheartening."

I said we would see him and his family as soon as possible. I suggested asking the ICU social worker to arrange a meeting with his family for one thirty, two hours from our conversation. Judith agreed. I was working that day with John Mecchella, a senior internal medicine resident. We briefly examined Daren and reviewed the orders and nursing notes to make sure that he was receiving sufficient medication for pain and anxiety. This is particularly important when a patient is paralyzed and, therefore, not only unable to speak but even unable to wince, stiffen, or furrow a brow to indicate discomfort. The doses of both made us confident that he was comfortable. No changes were needed. We spoke with his nurse, Anna, who agreed that he was very likely insensate and said that her main current concern was his respiratory status. The vent settings were as high as they could go and his oxygen levels were marginal.

We then met his parents, Marilyn and Daniel, his grandmother, his sister, Misty, and Uncle Ted, his mother's brother. Ted had just arrived from Panama where he is stationed as a civilian contractor for the U.S. military.

While the events replayed in my memory, in real time, Antonia projected salient points and a few quotes extracted from the Palliative Care Service consultation, including notes of the family meeting that Dr. Mecchella and I had entered in Daren's medical record.

Under the "reason for consultation" line in our consultation template we entered:

Family support in coping with their 25 year old son who is dying.

Under a "family meeting" header, we said that a meeting was convened in the ICU conference room that involved Daren's parents, sister, grandmother, and uncle, and included his nurse and the ICU social worker. We wrote:

Patient's family is trying to cope with the severity of his illness and the fact that he has been getting worse over the past few days. The family is aware of his very poor prognosis and the high likelihood that he will die from this. They want to be hopeful that he may recover, but are attempting to prepare for his death. They will be calling in additional friends and family who would like to come see Daren.

Under "CPR status," we wrote:

Has been Full Code. We discussed limitations of components of
CPR. Following discussion, family requested partial DNR status. Will allow vasopressors, but not allow chest compressions or
shocks.

These were the key points. Reading the excerpted notes on Antonia's
PowerPoint slide, I was drawn back to that day in the ICU meeting room.

After going around the table with brief introductions, I asked them
to talk about Daren as a person. They described a young man who was
generally happy and well adjusted. He was warm and loving, yet in style,
reserved, and private. He enjoyed his job and seemed poised to rise in
his company but, unless asked, rarely spoke about his work. During his
freshman year in high school Daren had told his parents that he was gay.
It was never a source of contention or even apparent discomfort within
his family.

He had a life away from his family, geographically and otherwise.
He loved to travel and did so with a circle of close male friends whom
his family knew by first names only. The exception was his sister, Misty,
who spoke up during the meeting to say that she had met several of
his friends during a four-day trip to Minneapolis in which she slept on
her brother's couch. She commented with a small smile, "By the way,
my brother also likes to party." This made his parents and Ted chuckle
because it was in contrast to Daren's reserved demeanor.

We discussed his course to date and their understanding of his current condition. They fully understood that the situation appeared grave.
Dr. Gladstone and the critical care team had broached the subject of
placing a tracheostomy, since it appeared that mechanical ventilation
might be needed for a longer term and it would be gentler for his windpipe. The team also raised the question of placing a PEG tube during
the same trip to the operating room.

Emotionally, his parents described being on a roller coaster that began in the Infectious Disease office and continued until Daren was emergently reintubated four days ago. It was an involuntary ride in which their hopes rose with every bit of good news and fell precipitously with every load of bad news. Now the ride had suddenly ended, the roller coaster collapsed, and tons of debris lay atop them. The weight of their grief made it hard for them to take a full breath. They were in despair.

We asked about their thoughts regarding the tracheostomy and PEG tube. They said they felt unprepared to make those decisions and would need a few days to think about it. I sensed they were annoyed that we had ever asked. Their unspoken reasoning was that Daren might not survive to benefit from the procedures, so why put him through them. Their hope was not completely gone, but drop by drop, with each new test result and complication—the infections, the IRIS, the pneumothoraces and blood clots—it kept leaking away. They were walking a fine tightrope, balancing any chance that Daren could still survive against a commitment to let him go if he could not survive. They clung to a statement from Dr. Hal Manning, a senior pulmonologist, who had said that if Daren did ultimately recover, his lungs would be damaged, but he did not think he would be a respiratory cripple. However, now that, too, seemed irrelevant because he was dying.

Marilyn and Daniel McCallum were reeling from the impending loss of their son. The weight of their grief was made worse by their ongoing commitment to keep tight the circle of family and friends who knew of Daren's condition.

My most vivid memory from that meeting was of Uncle Ted. When he introduced himself, Ted explained that he and Daren had always been close. Although it had taken Ted fifteen hours of travel to reach our hospital in Lebanon, New Hampshire, yesterday, he had spent the entire night in Daren's ICU room. He was a large, lean, and tanned man in his late forties with short, clipped light brown hair and a light blue shirt.

As we discussed Daren's condition and I asked if his family members felt Daren was comfortable, Ted related what he had seen and heard overnight.

He said he watched each laboratory blood draw, every arterial blood gas, and witnessed every time the nurses suctioned Daren's endotracheal tube. He said the gurgling of Daren's secretions being vacuumed up sent chills through his spine. Ted was subdued and spoke in a soft down-to-earth tone of someone earnestly attentive and thoroughly exhausted. Suddenly, however, his monotone was punctuated by an uncontrollable sob. The first time, he erupted in mid-sentence, while reporting what he had seen on the ICU monitor above the head of Daren's bed.

"His heart rate jumped about fifteen points each time he was suctioned"—Ted paused for a moment, recollecting his thoughts, then, without warning, let out a loud, keening wail, "oooHHH," followed by a staccato, involuntary in-breath: "huh-huh-HUH," and these followed by a low-pitched, mournful "Ohhhh." As soon as the wail passed, he continued—". . . and whenever they turned him in bed," determined to complete his report.

"Sorry, I just need a moment," he continued, apologizing for the interruption, but not for showing his emotions. It happened three more times as he spoke in an otherwise calm voice. Each time he cried, his body heaved in sea swells of grief, then, as the wave passed, he regained composure.

Marilyn reached over and took her brother's upper arm, shaking it softly. Smiling through tears she said, "You were not supposed to lose it. We needed you here to be strong for me!" Her teasing was gentle and her support strong. He placed his hand over hers and squeezed it but looked straight ahead. It was taking all his attention to maintain equilibrium.

We spent a significant portion of the meeting talking about ways that Daren's family members could take care of one another. The major decisions were made and goals of care clear. We would stay the course, but not further escalate treatment. With Daren basically asleep and on a

ventilator, receiving antimicrobials for his multiple infections and blood
thinners for the clots, his vital signs were being continuously monitored.
The curare-like medication was discontinued, so his level of comfort
was being carefully observed by the ICU nurses. It was time to turn
attention to his family.

They had moved into "vigil mode," staying in the hospital's cramped
waiting rooms, cafeteria, and public spaces when they were not directly
at Daren's bedside. I went through a list of the most basic things that
they each needed to do every day for their own well-being: at least a few
hours of sleep each day, some good food, some exercise and fresh air. We
reviewed, particularly for newcomers Ted and Misty, where they could
take showers if they felt unable to leave for the night.

I asked, "How are you doing within yourselves?" gesturing to my
chest as I spoke.

Daren's mother and father spoke of the emotional weight that keeping his condition confidential was adding to their situation. There were
two other sets of aunts and uncles, at least two other cousins and close
friends who would want to see Daren before he died. We discussed
Daren's desire for privacy. They believed that when Daren said those
things he assumed he was going to get well. His parents and sister felt
that if Daren knew that he was now likely to die, he would relax those
restrictions.

I offered another perspective that supported the same conclusion.
As much as Daren's survival and well-being were the focus for us all, he
was not the only one with a personal stake in this tragic situation. He
could constrain all of us on staff at the hospital from telling others about
his illness, but those restrictions did not apply to his family.

Medical ethics addresses when and how information can be shared
by doctors and other health care providers, as well as how it can be communicated to others, such as employers, insurance companies, relatives,
friends, and even law enforcement. But family rules are influenced by
culture and history of relationships. When a patient's mother or father

or siblings have information about a patient, they are not bound by the same rules. What is right will differ from one family to another and one situation to another. In listening to the history of Daren's relationships with his aunts and uncles and a few cousins and college friends, I felt confident it was reasonable for them to share the news of his critical condition and impending death with a wider, but still small, circle of close friends and family. I used my doctorly role to give them permission to do so.

Daren's condition changed little over the next several days. His parents did call a select group of relatives and friends, and the ranks of Daren's family vigil rose in the days that followed. I rotated off our hospital consultation service but continued to receive updates at our morning team meetings. Our team and volunteers visited daily. They brought a small "boom box" and CDs with music that Daren enjoyed. Karen Grocholski, our chaplain, brought a shawl that had been knitted by another group of volunteers and also visited daily, checking in on Daren and his parents to lend an ear and help in any way possible.

At forty-five minutes into her M&M, Antonia projected summary slides with data from day 1 through day 72 with bar graphs detailing the status of each of his conditions over time, his blood counts, including titers of viral load and number of CD4 cells. His HIV infection was responding to treatment. It looked like HIV wouldn't kill him—at least not directly—but his prognosis remained bleak. The cause of death would likely be a combination of the inflammatory syndrome or any one of his multiple viral and bacterial infections. A tracheostomy was performed and a PEG tube was placed. For days his ventilator settings remained maximally high, with pressures that threatened to rupture new blebs in his lungs.

A social worker's note in the chart captured the mood.

Met with patient's parents, Daniel and Marilyn, at his bedside. They were each holding one of his hands, mother talking to Daren in a soothing voice, assuring him that he is safe in their care and that anything that looked frightening was a side effect of his medications. She feels he is having hallucinations that are frightening him. Patient did look into his mother's eyes when she spoke and would then frequently close his eyes for a few moments. Several times during my visit, his eyes fixed on the ceiling, and his hands trembled. His mother's words brought his focus back to her and his hands relaxed.

The social worker's note continued.

I asked his parents how they are getting through this, to which his father stated that he believes they are "simply numb at this point." He and Marilyn cannot identify a source of strength or comfort for themselves today. They both note that they are very tired. They have a lot of trouble getting up in the morning. They just don't want to come in here and face this.

In the mind of the M&M audience, the only remaining question concerned how Daren died.

"And then," Antonia announced, "the clinical course took a surprising turn. Before concluding this case, I would like to introduce three guests at today's conference."

She pointed to the upper left corner of the lecture hall and said, "Please join me in welcoming Daren McCallum, and his parents, Marilyn and Daniel."

A thin, healthy-appearing young adult man dressed in black slacks and a pressed white shirt rose from his chair and smiled tentatively. To his right his parents beamed. People audibly gasped. The hall erupted in applause and people rose to their feet.

I have been to hundreds of M&M conferences and never saw anything remotely approaching this. I don't think there was a dry eye in the place.

When the stirring diminished, Antonia spoke again. The rest of the story, she explained, was exciting, yet easily told. On hospital day 96 his ventilator settings began to improve, slowly at first, and more quickly over the next two days. Concurrently, his blood counts improved and his chest X-rays showed signs of clearing. The IRIS had finally subsided; with the HAART drugs killing the HIV, his immune system began to recover and the other antiviral and antibiotic medications started to wipe out the other foreign invaders. The ICU team was able to lighten his sedation. As he became alert, Daren was able to follow instructions and even try short periods of time disconnected from the ventilator. Within another two days, he was able to tolerate having the ventilator disconnected for four and then eight hours at a time. Within a week he was extubated, the chest tubes were out, he was eating, and he was working with a physical therapist three hours a day without the need for extra oxygen. On hospital day 124 he was discharged to a rehabilitation facility, where he stayed for just a week before going home to his parents' house.

Between the day of his discharge and the M&M conference he had gained back eighteen of the twenty-two pounds he had lost. He was still taking HAART and blood-thinning medications but no longer taking antibiotics. His CD4 count was normal and his viral HIV load undetectable. He was as close to fully cured as a person with HIV can be.

Daren's survival is truly miraculous. It is thrilling for all of us who were involved in his care. Even a few years ago, Daren would surely have died from the collapse of his immune system and one or more of the opportunistic infections that resulted, his respiratory failure, or the blood clots in his lungs. Considering the virology and genomics of the HIV virus, the pharmacology of antiretroviral treatments, and the computing and imaging marvels of CT and MRI scanning, the amount of sheer science and technology involved in saving Daren rivals that required to send a man to the moon and back.

We rightly celebrate medical miracles of this magnitude. While recognizing our good fortune to live in the times we do, we would be wise to acknowledge the unprecedented challenges to clinical decision-making that these lifesaving advances represent.

Daren defied the odds. After he was reintubated and on maximal ventilator settings, the majority of the doctors and nurses caring for him thought he would die. Time was working against him. When one counts up factors that predict recovery for ICU patients, number of days in the ICU turns out to be a potent predictor of prognosis. In general, the longer a seriously injured or ill person requires a ventilator to breathe, the less well they do in the long run. At one academic center, a one-year follow-up of all ICU patients who survived more than twenty-one days of mechanical ventilation found that 44 percent of patients had died, 21 percent were fully dependent on others including paid caregivers, 26 percent were moderately dependent, and only 9 percent were fully independent in their daily functioning. Better outcomes tend to occur early. Daren was clearly an exception.

Daren's story illuminates an essential tension that clinicians, patients, and families are encountering as they strive to make sound medical decisions in life-threatening situations. It is the tension between making full use of lifesaving medical science and technology, while making sure people are comfortable and allowed to die gently when their time comes.

Stated most generally the question is: How can we derive full benefits from the unprecedented power that medical science and technology offer, while remembering that we have not made even one person immortal? In each case, the "how" will be highly specific to the person's individual values and preferences, as well as the particulars of their medical condition and available treatments. But the need to balance disease treatments with a recognition that each life will someday end is universal. If we are mortal, at some point in the course of illness, more treatment will not equal better care. But when?

There is no formula to apply and no facile way to make sound decisions. Wrestling with a decision is what makes it strong.

Reliable data about prognosis can inform physicians and help in

guiding seriously ill patients and their families through difficult decisions. I frequently refer to data when counseling people who are working
through difficult and often complex decisions about treatments. However, even when presented in plain speak and in context, the extent to
which historical population data can properly inform a specific patient's
situation is always open to question. Caution is warranted in applying
data from events that have happened to a unique, still-unfolding story.

For instance, if Daren were categorized as a ventilator-dependent
patient with a nontrauma medical condition, evidence from population
studies could easily be interpreted as predicting he would not survive.
A decision to withdraw the ventilator based on that data would not have
been wrong in any ethical or moral sense. Yet knowing what we know
now, it would have been dead wrong because, if acted upon, Daren
would have died.

It had taken 139 days in the hospital, just over half of them in the
ICU, during which Daren had more than five hundred laboratory tests,
fifty-seven blood cultures, 132 chest X-rays, one MRI, six CT scans, five
echocardiograms, two bronchoscopies, and a chest operation to sew up
blebs in his lungs. Seventeen clinical teams were involved in his care.
The total charges for his hospital treatments came to $1,061,629.41.

If Daren had died, his story would surely have made heads shake at
the extreme waste of limited resources for what were ultimately futile
treatments. Retrospectively, Daren's care would have been proven futile
by his death. But while he was alive, he still had a fleeting chance. And in
this case, that fleeting chance came to pass.

On the spectrum of treatments for late-stage illness, it is sobering
and humbling to recognize that Daren's care might well have looked
ridiculous if he had died, but happily, as events unfolded, it now seems
utterly sublime.

Part Four

Real Doctoring
for the
Twenty-first
Century

6.

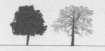

What Are Doctors For?

July 1 of the third year of medical school is the day the rubber hits the road, or rather, the day medical students hit the wards. On that day, they begin required rotations in internal medicine, surgery, pediatrics, obstetrics, and emergency medicine. After two years of studying anatomy, physiology, pharmacology, genetics, pathology, and other basic sciences, they don short white coats and start seeing patients. In so doing, students enter a new phase of training, an apprenticeship with roots deep in the antiquity of the profession.

Modern medicine is steeped in science, but still taught in the tradition of a craft within a guild community. In academic medical centers, third-year students occupy the first rung of the hierarchy of junior apprentice, journeyman, and master. Medical students are part observers, part scribes, and part "scut puppies." They run the errands, fill out the lab requests, and do routine chores that, well, someone has to do. They are usually happy to have scut work—medicalese for "some common unfinished tasks"—to do to feel useful. In return, students get to spend in-depth time with patients, taking histories, sometimes drawing blood for lab tests or assisting in bedside procedures, sometimes just visiting and supporting a patient. In addition, they get to be part of serious discussions among members of the team—their interns, residents, and attending physicians—about how best to care for seriously ill patients.

Medical students eagerly await their third year because, as anyone who has been through it knows, that is when you start to become a real doctor. You have been in school since age five and imagining being a doctor at least since college, and perhaps a lot longer. For two years of medical school, students have been relegated to classrooms and labs, or to being strictly observers of clinical care. Now, the pace of training quickens and in their third year medical students tend to grow up fast. The third year is at once exciting and scary; suddenly the things you have been reading about and watching, you are actually doing with— or *to*—real people. But students also feel the privilege—an earned privilege—of being present and involved in real medical care.

Medical students tend to look up to interns like they would big brothers and sisters. For interns—who were, themselves, medical students until July 1—taking on a teaching role can take some getting used to. Having graduated medical school, interns are doctors, but they are still a long way from being ready to practice independently. Interns are on a steep learning curve. While taking responsibility for patients' care, they closely rely upon—and if they are wise, adhere to—guidance from the residents and fellows who are at a stage in training to safely know what they are doing. Atop the professional ladder at academic medical centers are the faculty physicians: assistant, associate, and full professors. They occupy the position of masters of the guild and provide firm direction, oversight, and teaching.

By and large, it is a benevolent community and hierarchy.

Well-functioning teams are collegial, each person pulling his or her own weight and supporting one another in getting work done, dealing with urgencies and mishaps, and picking up slack when necessary. During my own third- and fourth-year clinical rotations, I was often bone tired, but I never felt oppressed. As a medical student and later as an intern, my respect for senior residents and attending physicians bordered on awe. They seemed to know everything and I was grateful they invested time in teaching me and very glad to have them look over my shoulder. If all this sounds romantic, it is merely a reflection of how passionately I wanted to learn to be a doctor. My clinical training was exhilarating—and I loved it—but it was also exhausting and sobering. I think of it as postdoctoral training in devastating medical and social problems and human suffering. Through it all, my older colleagues and faculty physicians taught and modeled good practice for me and enabled me to become a real doctor.

Medical students' passion for learning as much as they possibly can persists to the present day. And through all the unprecedented challenges to medical practice, generosity toward junior members of our profession pervades medical training.

Today, I am an attending physician in my fourth decade of clinical practice, ultimately responsible for the quality of care delivered by the team I supervise. Concomitantly, in my role as a faculty physician at a teaching hospital, I am responsible for furthering the education and professional development of each clinician-in-training on the team, and I strive to perpetuate this age-old spirit of generous collegiality.

Something else changes abruptly in the third year of medical school. Students who have worked, studied—and played—intensively together for two years, are suddenly flung apart. Classmates and good friends one has seen nearly every day for two years are now dispersed across myriad rotations, clinical teams, and several hospitals. It can be jarring.

Each November, Dartmouth Medical School brings third-year students back together for two weeks for a seminar class called ICE, which stands for Integrated Clinical Experience. The ICE course delves into crosscutting clinical and ethical topics that the preceding third-year class nominated for inclusion.

For several years running, palliative and end-of-life care have been among the topics chosen by students. Each November members of our team—one or more physicians, usually with a nurse practitioner, chaplain, or social worker—have been accorded four hours to discuss how we approach caring for people whom we cannot cure.

Four hours may not seem like much for so important a topic. It's not, but curriculum time is a precious commodity and those few hours are roughly a fifth of the total hours of course work that medical students have on these topics. So our team is determined to use the time well.

My two-hour session this day would challenge the students to explore how we can best serve seriously ill people and their families— and invite them to continue thinking deeply about these issues as they continue their training and enter their practices. The following day a physician colleague and social worker from our team would engage the students in practicing skills of communicating bad news and discussing with patients what treatments they would want, or not want, in life-threatening situations.

ICE is usually held in the medical school's Chilcott Auditorium, which fits the seventy-five or eighty students who are able to attend. (Inevitably a few are away on off-cycle clinical rotations.) Chilcott is a comfortable setting for lectures; acoustics and audiovisual equipment are fine, but it is less than ideal for group discussions. The auditorium is a terraced arc of seats facing down and center, where instructors stand at a podium or pace before a whiteboard, looking up at students who, these days, tend to stare at their laptops rather than at the person teaching. It can be hard to spark a genuine conversation.

This November's ICE class was scheduled for one p.m. and it was nearly eight minutes passed the hour before people took seats and began to settle. Knowing that our session would start after lunch, I planned to keep the lights on and the PowerPoint projector off, in hopes of keeping the students engaged.

I introduced myself briefly; most students knew me from a couple of lectures I gave during their first- and second-year courses. Additionally, at least a quarter of the class had already interacted with me or our team during clinical rotations at DHMC.

"I want to start by thanking you for including this topic in the ICE course again this year. Technically, my thanks belong to the senior class who chose this topic on your behalf. I am grateful and hope to earn your vote for these subjects to be included again next year.

"Secondly, I want to apologize to you. To this point in your training, we have not been preparing you as well as we should to care for seriously ill and dying patients, nor for the families who love, care, and worry about these patients day in and day out. I believe we have been setting you up to fail. It is not right and I am sorry."

Even the students who had not quite settled in, and those who had been quickly checking their e-mails, stopped and looked up.

"I speak solely for myself as one member of the faculty—and my faculty colleagues may take exception to my belief. So, the apology is my own. We have been gradually improving our curriculum at Dartmouth Medical School, but change has been incremental and slow in coming. To be fair, our school is hardly alone in underemphasizing topics and skills related to life-limiting conditions. I often ask the residents I work with—who as you know come to DHMC from a wide variety of medical schools across the country, and other countries—about their education in palliative aspects of care. Most feel they have not been adequately taught basic skills: How to give the bad news to a patient that her cancer has progressed, or tell a family a loved one has died. How to introduce hospice care to a patient and family. How to explain CPR in a way people can readily understand. Interns and residents may recall having one lecture on pain management and another on the ethics of stopping life-prolonging treatments. They don't feel competent to treat a patient's cancer-caused pain, nor are they confident in guiding decisions that allow for a patient to die naturally, or even how to encourage people to complete advance directives. Only a few say that they had good training and mentoring in these skills. (It is a mark of national progress that at least a few do.)

"Just for interest, let's take a quick straw poll of your collective plans for practice. How many people here plan to provide prenatal care and deliver babies in their practice?"

Three students raised their hands.

"How many plan to care for newborns?"

Four more hands went up.

"Thanks. And how many of you plan to specialize in one of the following: family medicine, internal medicine, cardiology, nephrology, neurology, oncology, pulmonology, anesthesiology, infectious disease, interventional radiology, radiation oncology, critical care, general surgery, or oncologic, thoracic, cardiovascular, or neurosurgery?"

All but eight hands went up.

"To those who just raised their hands, in each of your specialties a significant portion of the patients you will treat will be elderly. Many will have life-threatening conditions. Without a doubt, it will be common in your practices to examine, treat, and counsel people who go on to die. Whether you intend to or not, you will be providing end-of-life care."

No one was looking at laptops.

"Think about the hours of course work you have had on embryology, reproductive medicine, prenatal care, labor and delivery, and neonatal care—and about the four- to six-week rotations in obstetrics and pediatrics that are required in this third year. Now consider how many hours of required classes and clinical rotation are devoted to topics related to dying, caregiving, and grief?

"In this regard, as in most medical schools, our curriculum seems well suited to the 1940s and '50s when most doctors delivered babies and routinely took care of infants.

"Times have changed and health care has become highly specialized.

These days every doctor who plans to care for pregnant women or deliver babies has to complete a residency in either obstetrics or family medicine.

"And last time I checked, only 50 percent of the population is at risk of having an obstetrical experience in their lifetimes, while epidemiological studies continue to find that 100 percent of Americans eventually die."

That generated a laugh.

"Most medical schools do not require hospice or palliative care rotations, many do not even offer them as electives. Medical schools generally provide a lecture or two on pain management and discuss the ethics of end-of-life decisions and palliative and end-of-life topics within other courses. The total course content of these topics probably amounts to fifteen to twenty-five hours over the four years of medical school curriculum."

I glanced at my watch, smiled drily, and said, "So, in the three hours and forty-seven minutes remaining to us, I am going to try to make up for these deficiencies."

All kidding aside, I had ambitious goals for my brief time with these students.

"First and foremost, I hope to give you a sense that caring well for people who are dying is not merely a responsibility—and it is—but also offers deeply meaningful therapeutic opportunities. I hope to provide you with a framework for being the best doctors you can be for patients who are seriously ill and for their families. My goal is to equip you to evaluate all you will see and hear in the years ahead about care for people through the end of life; to critically evaluate the science and clinical guidelines you will read in journals and learn in presentations, as well as the interactions and practice patterns of your teachers and colleagues that you will witness.

"If you understand what really excellent care through the end of life looks and *feels like*—to your patients and as their physician—you will be able to distinguish not just good care from bad care but what is truly first-rate from what is merely mediocre. With this discernment, you can continue learning from it all."

I paused. "That should suffice for the afternoon, eh?

"Okay, let's begin. Now that you have had a few months of concentrated clinical experience under your belts, I'd like to pose a simple question for discussion: What are doctors for?"

I picked up a marker and walked to the whiteboard in the front of the room while looking around the auditorium. No one said anything for the first ten or fifteen seconds.

"I can start, if you'd like." That was enough to break the ice.

"Saving lives," a small young woman in the back of the lecture hall said in a strong voice.

"Good," I replied. "Pretty much the prime directive, isn't it? We are here to save lives. No doubt about it. Would it be fair to say, as an extension of this principle, that doctors are for diagnosing and treating the things that ail us?"

I paused and panned the room. No one objected and several nodded in agreement.

"For most people, most of the time, our job description is to save life—cure disease, fix serious injuries, mend broken organs and limbs—and restore people to physical health.

"How about when we are unable to cure people? When a patient has a life-limiting illness or injury, what are doctors for, then?"

"We can treat pain," one student spoke out.

"Absolutely." I wrote TREATING PAIN on the whiteboard and said, "If you'll allow me, I would expand this bullet to say, TREATING PAIN & ALLE-VIATING SUFFERING. We still can't cure many diseases, including many cancers, but we can always diminish pain and alleviate suffering.

"We may not be able to completely *relieve* a person's suffering—not all physical discomfort and certainly not all emotional and existential distress can be resolved—but we can always make a person's distress at least a little less severe, a little easier for a patient to tolerate."

I planned to spend about a half hour defining categories and writing bullet points on the whiteboard as the students explored various ways doctors can help people living with incurable conditions and facing the end of life. I was about to move on when a woman in the second row with short, red hair and an expression that telegraphed consternation raised her hand.

As I acknowledged her, she said, "Dr. Byock, I hear what you are saying, but I don't think pain is all that well treated. I've had two rotations—surgery and neurology—in which I have seen patients whose pain wasn't controlled at all. One woman had metastatic lung cancer and had emergency neurosurgery to drain an intracerebral hemorrhage. Our team saw her at least twice every day. She had terrible back and hip pain from her cancer—and had been taking high doses of pain medicine before her bleed—but they would only give her Tylenol. She asked for more pain medication every time I saw her. One time she squeezed my hand and said, 'Why won't you help me?' It was awful. I told our resident and he spoke with the attending on rounds. But we were told, 'We have to follow her mental status.'"

I sighed, reminding myself that examples of what not to do can be as valuable in teaching as examples to emulate.

"Obviously, I do not know the details of this case beyond what you have just described. I don't want to second-guess or unfairly criticize my fellow faculty physicians. However, I can say that it is not necessary to withhold pain medications in order to accurately follow people's mental status. If that is what that attending physician believes, I strongly disagree. Particularly in older patients, uncontrolled pain can cause mental confusion and even florid delirium. In one study of patients undergoing hip surgery, elders without dementia who were in severe pain after surgery had nine times the risk of becoming delirious, compared to patients whose pain was properly treated with morphine. The take-home lesson is that when pain is carefully treated and closely monitored, people's minds usually remain clear.

"There is a famous aphorism in medicine: 'To cure sometimes, to relieve often, to comfort always.' 'To comfort always' does not apply only to patients with advanced disease. When I was in medical school, we were taught that it was unfortunate, but necessary, for patients being evaluated for possible appendicitis or gallbladder attack to go without pain treatment in order for physicians to accurately monitor sequential abdominal examinations. Since then, surgery and emergency medicine studies have proven that that is not true. Patients with a hotly inflamed gallbladder or appendix still tightened their abdominal muscles to guard from a physician's examining hand, and patients with peritonitis still have 'rebound tenderness' when a doctor palpates and releases pressure on their abdomens. By being more comfortable, patients are better able to cooperate with doctors, who are, in turn, better able to perform adequate physical examinations. Simply put, allowing someone to be in severe pain is not good medicine."

I continued, wanting to provide tangible support to the student who asked the question and to any others who have had—or will have—similar experiences.

"In contemporary medical practice if the steps at managing pain or other sources of suffering are not successful, there are always additional things we can try. During your rotations at DHMC, if pain is particularly difficult to control, you can always call the Acute Pain Service for help. Or if the patient has an advanced illness and either pain or a constellation of symptoms that is complex, our Palliative Care Service team is available to answer questions or see a patient in consultation at any time."

I paused before making the next point.

"I understand that the attending physician in charge has to allow you or our team to formally request a consultation from the Pain Service or Palliative Care, but the large majority of them will. If not, enlist the help of the patient's nurses. You have probably already picked up on a timeless truth that medical students and interns know: when a direct approach fails, nurses can almost always get the consultation."

A few students chuckled and more than a few heads nodded in agreement.

Turning back to the student who asked the question, I said, "I appreciate the example; I wish I could say it was rare. Throughout the rest of your training you will learn from your teachers' positive examples, and their occasional shortcomings. As I said, my purpose today is to sharpen your discernment. It is an important part of lifelong learning."

I scanned the room. People seemed ready to proceed.

"Okay, let's move on. What else are doctors for?"

A lanky male student on my right, seated near the back of the room, raised his hand and spoke. "Doctors give people information about their health and about treatments for their medical problems."

"Right. We give information. A key reason that we give information is to teach people about their health. As you probably know, the Latin root of the word 'doctor' is *docere*, meaning 'to teach.'

"We give people information about their medical condition and treatment options. We provide and make sense of technical information in the process of helping people make critical decisions. The term and concept in vogue these days is shared decision-making—the process by which doctors and patients work together in coming to sound decisions. We also can give patients and their families information about their prognoses, their chances for recovery, and what their capacities and needs will likely be in the future.

"Our role as a key source of reliable information and teaching continues through the end of life. As people's conditions change, they continually need pertinent information about their condition and treatments, and help with learning how to take good care of themselves."

The conversation continued for a while. Students asked questions about differences in communicating with patients with various diagnoses—cancer, heart failure, liver failure, and ALS (amyotrophic lateral sclerosis). We talked about the ways that quality of life, risks, and potential benefits of treatments all weigh into making sound decisions.

I felt we were making good use of our time, but if I was going to help these young doctors-to-be become all they could be, I needed to sail into deeper water.

"Is ending people's lives one of the things that doctors are for?"

I paused again and looked around the room. A couple of people's heads nodded, two or three shook a "no," and a few cocked one ear in my direction, as if listening for an echo of the question. No student spoke.

"I'm not going to ask for a show of hands. I assume there are people in the room on both sides of the assisted suicide debate. Some of you will practice in states in which physician-assisted suicide is legal, or will become legal.

"Today's discussion is not intended to be political, though we can't ignore the fact that this political and social controversy can impact our clinical practice. In full disclosure, I have written and spoken against bills and referendums to make physician-assisted suicide legal. And I remain firmly opposed. However, several years ago I came to the conclusion that both sides—pro and con—are wrong and dropped out of the fight. My purpose today is to stay focused on clinical principles that can help you become the best physicians you can be and help you give people who are seriously ill the best care possible."

The room was still. But the students were clearly engaged. So far, so good. I'd budgeted about twenty-five minutes for this discussion. I am keenly aware that the issue of assisted suicide is not just a hot political topic but a source of confusion and doubt in many physicians' minds. Many lay people and more than a few doctors conflate intensive management of suffering or stopping life-sustaining treatments with euthanasia. It was worth investing the time to draw clear distinctions.

"It's worth considering another question. Is it necessary to end some dying people's lives in order to relieve their suffering?"

They recognized my question to be rhetorical: I was the only gray-haired, practicing physician in the room.

"I can say this: I have never willfully allowed a patient to die suffering. And in over thirty years of practice in hospice and palliative care, I have never found it necessary to euthanize a patient."

I spoke in an unhurried manner so that the students could consider, absorb, or reject my assertions.

"To be sure, there have been plenty of patients whom I made sleepy with medications and some I rendered fully unconscious to ensure they were not suffering as they died. Some people ask, 'Well, what's the difference between that and euthanasia?' Most concretely, the difference is that I have never injected potassium chloride to stop someone's heart or given curare to stop a person's breathing and cause a person's death."

I explained the critical clinical and moral distinction between killing a patient and letting the person die. Except in the midst of acute rescue efforts for casualties at the scene of an accident, or performing CPR on a previously vital victim of a sudden cardiac arrest, there comes a time in every life when it is acceptable to let a person die.

"Most people's pain, air hunger, or anxious distress can be alleviated with medications that are, or will become, familiar to you: opioids, benzodiazepines, and the phenothiazine family of drugs. With good care, most people are relatively comfortable and interactive until the last days and sometimes hours of life. It would be great if it were possible to make every patient comfortable and alert. Research into novel pain treatments and medications may one day make this a reality. For now, sometimes being drowsy is the cost of being comfortable.

"Many of the patients and families we care for may not clearly distinguish *letting die* from *ending life.* On occasion a relative of an ICU patient who is unresponsive and having his or her life maintained has quietly confided to me, 'We put dogs out of their misery' or 'This is why I believe in Dr. Kevorkian.' I recognize the grief in such comments, yet am struck by a certain irony. It is true that we sometimes euthanize sick dogs and cats, but primarily we do not put them on ventilators or kidney dialysis machines and infuse vasopressor medications into them in ICUs. Instead, we allow them to die naturally.

"The people Jack Kevorkian euthanized were not being kept alive moment-to-moment by medical machines. If they had been, their doctors could have turned them off.

"The point I want to make is this: *Alleviating suffering* and *eliminating the sufferer* are very different acts."

Doctors need to understand these distinctions. There are no clinical or ethical restrictions to alleviating pain when someone is dying. The established ethical principle of double effect allows for an unintended harm—including a person's death—to occur while striving toward a good. High-risk surgery may be performed in the hope of saving a person's life, or high-dose pain and sedative medications administered to relieve a person's suffering. In neither situation does a patient's death constitute killing; acting with the intention of shortening a person's life does.

So much of medicine carries caveats, exceptions, and ambiguities. Particularly in the realm we were discussing, I wanted to give the students simple, unambiguous guidelines whenever possible.

"I really meant what I said earlier about alleviating suffering." I pumped my thumb in the direction of the TREATING PAIN & ALLEVIATING SUFFERING bullet on the whiteboard.

"We will encounter people whose lives we cannot save—diseases we cannot cure and injuries too grave to repair—but we can *always* make dying people more comfortable. As the priorities of a patient's care shifts from quantity of life to quality of life, comfort becomes paramount. When someone is dying, any concerns about long-term side effects of medications or addiction to narcotic pain relievers are unwarranted."

Okay. Now that I had led the class into deep water, it was time to throw them a line.

"If all of this seems overwhelmingly complex or daunting right now, please don't worry. As long as you have the interest, you will find caring for people through the end of life to be a natural extension of the knowledge and clinical skills you are already developing. Excellent care for people who are dying needs to be meticulous, methodical, proactive, and ongoing with regard to managing symptoms, conversations, and planning, but it is usually fairly straightforward.

"When specialists are needed, these days there are palliative care consultants to call in. As you go through your training, remember this: there is no ethical, physiologic, or pharmacologic reason today for any person to die in agony. On the contrary, allowing someone to die suffering is medically and ethically wrong."

A student on the left side of the room raised his hand, hesitated, and then started to speak. "I have read and thought a lot about these issues. I agree with most of what you have said, but I guess I feel that dying people have a right to do what they want with their own bodies."

"This is partially true," I said. "I appreciate your comment. A number of ethics commissions, including the Presidential Commission for the Study of Bioethical Issues, and seminal court decisions, have said that people have a right to refuse any medical treatments that are offered and must be given a chance to decide among legitimate and available treatments for their conditions. If they are of sound mind—meaning have 'decision-making capacity'—people can refuse antibiotics for pneumonia or urinary sepsis, so-called 'feeding tubes,' or even insulin if they are diabetic, knowing full well that they will die without treatment.

"But the commissions, blue-ribbon panels, and the courts have also said that people do not have a right to receive any treatments they desire. The responsibility for determining what treatment options are indicated and presenting those options to patients rests firmly with physicians. A patient might dearly want a heart transplant or a stem cell transplant for leukemia, but be ineligible because of coexisting conditions. A patient with widely metastatic melanoma may want neurosurgery for a cerebral lesion, but if the consulting neurosurgeon deems that the procedure is not in the patient's best interest, she can refuse to perform the operation. Similarly, physicians need not perform CPR on a patient if the procedure would be literally futile.

"Consistent with this principle, most courts, legislatures, and ethics commissions have concluded that people do not have the authority to demand and receive from doctors legal medications intended to end their lives. But it feels incomplete to respond to your question solely from the perspective of rights. I want to refocus on the question I first posed: What are doctors for?

"Even if society deems it legal—for purposes of criminal liability and life insurance—for dying people to commit suicide, the medical profession believes—as do I—that intentionally ending a person's life is beyond the scope of medicine."

I explained that although I remain firmly opposed to society legalizing assistance with suicide, I believe it would be less erosive to physicians' roles and patients' trust if proponents kept doctors out of the process. After all, our expertise is needed only to certify that a person who desires the means for ending his or her life actually has a terminal condition. The doses of drugs used to hasten death do not vary by age or weight. Instead of a doctor's prescription, responsibility for issuing permission to a certified patient to purchase a packet of lethal medications could be assigned to another civic authority, such as the county attorney or justice of the peace. I'd still vote against a referendum on such a policy, but compared to physician-assisted suicide, this approach would mitigate damage to the social architecture. It would leave doctors free to focus on alleviating suffering and improving quality of patients' lives.

"I worry about the social and cultural consequences of doctors ending lives," I concluded.

"I understand," he said. "I am going to have to think about this more."

"Very well. Of course, you have the right—and, for what it's worth, my permission—to disagree. Thanks again for the comment," I replied.

"We still have a few minutes before we take a break. We are already

uicide. I hadn't planned to, but

couple of steps further in the

o objection and more than a

rspective, any serious request

ler life must be seen as a red

fering or fears uncontrollable
future suffering. 'Doctor, will you help me die?' should be considered
an impending medical emergency until proven otherwise, much like a
patient who says, 'Doctor, I have a squeezing pain, right here,'" I said,
holding my clenched right fist over my heart. "Until you are a senior resident, such statements will always require evaluation by someone more
experienced. Not all such requests turn out to be emergencies. 'Doctor,
will you help me die?' may be the way a person asks for assurance that
she will not be in severe pain as she dies—perhaps like her mother or
father in the last hours of life. At very least, such questions are opportunities to listen and respond to a person's worst fears."

I explained that in their next year's seminar course we would discuss
ways of responding to such requests that can reassure patients, build
trust, and be therapeutically effective. And I encouraged them to consider taking an elective rotation with our Palliative Care Service during
their fourth year.

"A moment ago, I said there was a distinction between suicide and
assisted suicide. In my experience, seriously ill people who are hurting
and scared usually already have the means to end their lives. People
with cancer or heart, liver, lung, or kidney disease usually have cabinets
or drawers full of prescription medications for pain, sleep, or anxiety
that, when taken in combination with alcohol, will provide a swift and
painless exit. Websites provide information on ways to do the job with
tools as available as a car in a garage.

"People who feel helpless and hopeless frequently have the means, but may be asking for their doctor's prescription to find out whether their doctor *agrees* they are helpless and without hope. From a therapeutic perspective, doctors must steadfastly stand for helping and hoping for a better quality of life."

I wanted to peel the onion of this topic another layer and invite them to consider the psychology of a physician's decision to assist or not to assist a terminally ill patient in ending his or her life.

"When a doctor cannot think of anything else to do for someone who is suffering, assisted suicide or even euthanasia may look like the right thing to do.

"You probably already have had a taste of how a doctor's emotional state might influence this. If the doctor has had a long, hard stretch of being on call or a series of difficult cases, it is easy to understand how his or her own distress might contribute to a sense of feeling overwhelmed and constrain effective counseling or identification of viable therapeutic options.

"In fact, the decision to assist in preempting death may respond to the doctor's suffering as much as to the patient's fears or suffering. Proponents of legalizing physician-assisted suicide object when I say this, but I mean it with all humility.

"Dr. Robert Twycross, a venerable British physician and professor of palliative medicine at Oxford University, has written that 'a doctor who has never been tempted to kill a patient probably has had limited clinical experience or is not able to empathize with those who suffer.'

"I have met many patients over the years that I thought would be better off if they were to die soon. I have been tempted to end more than one suffering person's life. That is precisely why our profession has developed formal standards of practice and statements of ethical practice—to remind us that such acts are wrong."

Again I paused and looked around the auditorium. This key point warranted the time.

"We are just human beings bringing special expertise to bear to serve others. We have feelings and are prone to stress and exhaustion, and even burnout. That is one reason why we work in teams. And that is why these days, in all academic centers and most large hospitals, we have palliative medicine specialists working within palliative care teams to call on for help. Effectively treating complex pain and counseling people with profound emotional suffering is difficult, time- and labor-intensive, and emotionally draining. Even the best doctors benefit from the perspective, knowledge, and skills of nurses, social workers, chaplains, pharmacists, and others.

"In case you haven't yet noticed, doctors often get very attached to their patients. Truth be told, doctors often love patients. The warm positive regard that doctors feel for patients is wholesome and ethical. Codes of conduct and statements of professional practice serve as external checks when our feelings—pain or elation—threaten to sway our sound judgment.

"Like the cement foundation and I beams of a building, professional guidelines maintain the structural integrity of our profession through difficult times—including wars, economic depressions, natural disasters, and other social turmoil. From earliest antiquity, one professional boundary has been clear: doctors must not intentionally kill patients. This boundary is valid today, even in states and countries where the practice is legal. Our profession has consistently asserted other boundaries, sometimes against political pressures. It is, for instance, legal, but firmly unethical, for doctors to perform state-sanctioned executions. Even in times of war, doctors must refrain from using medical skills to inflict pain on prisoners. Right?"

Again, as I panned the hall, students were taking this in, no doubt deciding how much of what I said they agreed or disagreed with. A number of students were leaning forward on folded arms or elbow. Several heads bobbed in agreement.

"We live in a world in which resources are limited and suffering abounds, in which comprehensive care is costly and hard to come by and lethal prescriptions are cheap. Even today, when many emergency departments and hospitals are filled to overflowing with people who have fallen through our frayed social safety net, I worry "self-deliverance" is another expedient way for society to avoid the costs and the messy complexities of actually providing excellent medical treatments along with authentic person- and family-centered care.

"Whether you are in favor of legalizing physician-assisted suicide or not—and whether assisting in suicide is legal where you practice or not—let's not allow our profession to become society's answer to suffering and the high costs of dying.

"Having formal professional guidelines that clearly define what can and cannot be done can be liberating, rather than confining, in one's practice. I have never had to abandon a patient who wanted to die at a time of his or her own choosing. By clarifying that I cannot and will not write lethal prescriptions, I have been able to avoid entangled negotiations, while unequivocally affirming my commitment to treat pain, alleviate suffering, and improve the quality of the person's life.

"Okay. Once again, please feel free to disagree. As the song goes, 'you take what you need and leave the rest.'

"Let's break for ten minutes. When we come back I promise to lighten things up a bit and talk about imagination, friendship, and the many things we can do for people facing the end of life."

When we reconvened, I began again. "To this point, our exploration of what doctors are for in serving people who are seriously ill has been pretty ponderous and heavy. At least some of you must be wondering why the heck I would choose to practice palliative medicine. In fact, caring for people through late stages of illness and through the end of their lives is the most satisfying and personally rewarding practice I have ever had.

"Doctors have existed in every society and culture to accompany patients on their journey through illness and death. Doctors have special skills and expertise to bring to the relationship. Whatever else I cannot do therapeutically, I can skillfully, confidently accompany the person who is ill for at least part of his or her journey.

"Although I am wary of overstretching metaphors, thinking of illness as an unwanted journey has been a useful way for me to explain my relationship to patients and their families. I may only see a patient and family for a short phase of their experience with illness but, like a captain of a passenger liner or the pilot of a plane, for the time they are in my charge my goal is to provide the best service possible.

"All the categorical things that doctors are for that we mentioned earlier fit nicely within this illness-as-journey concept. If you are a doctor accompanying someone on a journey—perhaps backpacking or rafting—and the person becomes hurt and is in pain, of course you are going to do what you can to make the person comfortable. If your companion develops a medical problem with which you are skilled in managing, naturally you would offer your advice and assistance.

"In thinking about the process of dying as a metaphorical journey, additional doctorly responsibilities and therapeutic opportunities come into view. Doctors can provide guidance for what lies ahead. On any journey with another person, if you know that a path widens and offers safe passage, naturally you are going to suggest taking it. If, however, you have previously traveled a road and know it becomes impassable a few miles ahead, naturally you are going to advise that you and your companion take a different route.

"Pediatricians refer to 'anticipatory guidance' in teaching parents of young infants what to expect and prepare for in the days, weeks, and months ahead. The concept applies well to the end of life. People commonly feel unprepared and at a loss in knowing how to get through this difficult, frightening, and often treacherous stretch in their and their family's lives. Doctors come to know where the hazards lie, what to watch out for, what to do before people are too much further along. We come to know how people can best prepare for these difficult, unwanted, yet common life events."

At the break a student had asked me when and how to bring up advance directives with patients. These topics were going to be covered in the next day's session. Two of the faculty members from our palliative care team—Dr. Annette Macy and our social worker, Laura Rollano—would be engaging the students in exercises to practice these conversations. But I wanted to introduce the subject here.

"A word about advance directives: I advise every adult to have an advance directive. The earlier in the illness journey it is completed, the better. Occasionally, surgeons or oncologists who have heard me make this point challenge me, saying that it is very hard for them to bring up advance directives with patients at the time of diagnosis or when they are just starting treatments. 'Ira,' they explain, 'that is when we are trying to build their hope.'

"The truth is, once a person is diagnosed, there is never a perfect time to bring up advance directives. It doesn't get easier when people begin having side effects of treatment, or when they have a complication such as a blood clot or infection that lands them in the hospital. It is not easy when their cancer progresses—hope is an even bigger deal then.

"There's a saying in palliative care: 'It's always too soon, until it's too late.' If a patient expresses concerns when you bring up advance directives—'But doctor, I thought you said you might be able to cure me!'—you need to be able to say two things: First: 'We ask *everybody* to complete advance directives, because we believe knowing who you would choose to speak for you and what your values and preferences are in case of life-threatening situations is important to providing you the best care possible.' Second, you need to be able to say: 'I have an advance directive, because I want the best health care for myself—and I want to support my family as much as I can if they are forced to make critical decisions about treatments for me.'"

I explained that, in our role as teachers, we can model that the optimal time for anyone to complete an advance directive is before it is needed.

"The single most effective way to prepare yourself to counsel patients about advance directives is to complete one yourself. Unless and until you do, it may feel awkward, a bit like a physician who smokes cigarettes counseling a patient on quitting, or a morbidly obese physician counseling a patient on weight loss."

A few students chuckled and I noticed that several students were talking to one another.

"Where can we get them, Dr. Byock?" a student asked.

"Dr. Macy and Laura Rollano will bring a pile of both New Hampshire and Vermont forms tomorrow morning for you to read and, hopefully, complete. It is part of the class exercise. You can also get them from several sites on the Internet."

I wasn't through with the illness-as-journey metaphor quite yet.

"When a patient is dying, accompanying entails walking with a person on a journey that ends in the person's death. Accompanying implies that we physicians will not abandon a person who makes a treatment decision with which we disagree. It may be that a patient refuses a treatment we think she really should have, or that a patient demands an operation or course of treatment that is not in her best interests. My consistent stance is: I am here to serve.

"But I need not relinquish my good judgment or sacrifice my professional integrity to continue this journey with a patient. In states where physician-assisted suicide is legal, not abandoning patients would entail continuing to care for people who had obtained a lethal prescription from other physicians. While I would not take part in the suicide, I would continue to *walk with* patients, alleviating the person's discomfort, optimizing his or her quality of life, and assisting the person to accomplish whatever he or she feels it is important to do before he or she dies."

I explained that professional boundaries are intended to protect and prevent doctors from acting in inappropriate or unprofessional ways. But professional boundaries on doctors' conduct are not meant to be emotional armor to prevent us from being authentic with patients.

"You are going to be practicing medicine for much of your waking life. If you can't be yourself during your working days—and nights—practice is going to feel pretty onerous."

"Many students and physicians-in-training believe that professional boundaries prohibit doctors from being friends with a patient. Not true.

"It is fully acceptable to be or become friends with a person who happens to be a patient. It is only natural for it to happen from time to time. In fact, if you practice in a small town—and I have practiced in a few—it's hard to avoid treating people who happen to be friends. Rural doctors inevitably end up caring for a few of their neighbors—as well as their lawyer or accountant or barber or beautician, or mechanics, or fellow congregants—patient-friends are nearly inescapable.

"Extending friendship to a patient invites true compassion, not merely sympathy or kindness but a willingness to suffer with the other. Authentic compassion on the part of a physician may entail expressing one's own feelings of frustration, disappointment, and sadness to a patient.

"At the same time, 'being real' implies being willing to say difficult things to patients when necessary.

"Patients are not the only ones who benefit when a doctor is able to be real. It is within authentic relationships with patients that the personal rewards of our profession are found."

It was time to illustrate these principles with a story from my own practice.

"Let me tell you about my friend Burt, a patient I met when the bone marrow transplant team asked us to help him with overwhelming anxiety associated with his illness and being confined to the hospital for long weeks at a time.

"Burt had myelodysplastic syndrome and unfortunately developed leukemia. In Burt's case, his only chance of being cured was a stem cell transplant. I explained to the students that the stem cell or bone marrow transplant patients are sometimes confined to their rooms for weeks or even months at a stretch. In preparation for the transplant, patients are given highly toxic chemotherapy and radiation treatments to sterilize their bone marrow and bloodstream of the diseased cells, as well as the healthy immune cells—lymphocytes and granulocytes—that would reject the newly transplanted cells.

"By killing all of their blood-forming cells—precursors of red cells, platelets, and the full gamut of white cells—people are rendered utterly vulnerable to bleeding and germs. Many develop infections and require daily doses of multiple intravenous antibiotics, plus antifungal and antiviral medications. It is common—even expected—for people to feel weak and sick to their stomachs. And it is normal for people to be worried about their future. With good reason. The list of complications that hematological transplant patients are prone to is long and scary. While stem cell and other bone marrow transplants have revolutionized treatment of childhood and many adult blood disorders, including leukemia, for adults receiving cells from unrelated donors, transplants are successful in less than half of cases. Sometimes even when 'successful,' the condition recurs months or years later. Still, for many people, the arduous process is all well worth going through because it offers a real chance for a cure.

"Burt wanted to live, but he was reeling from the physical and emotional assaults of his disease and its treatment. For him, being in the hospital before and after undergoing a stem cell transplant was a bit like going to jail—except a whole lot worse.

"When our team met him, Burt had been in the hospital for over a week. He was figuratively climbing the walls, although if his bad hip, the result of an old injury, hadn't hurt so much, he might have been climbing literally. As it was, he was tethered by a clutter of clear plastic tubes to two pumps and three IV bags clamped or hanging from a rolling steel stand. When he had the energy and his left hip wasn't aching, he paced around his room with that stand—a bit like a mouse on a wheel—but much of the time he was too exhausted and uncomfortable to walk farther than to and from his bathroom. So he spent long hours lying in bed.

"Burt was a tough, no-nonsense guy—at least that was the persona he cultivated. Within the first two minutes of meeting him, Burt would proudly and loudly tell you that he was a right-wing conservative and that 'Rush is right!' When tests and treatments allowed—or he wasn't puking—he listened faithfully to Rush Limbaugh, watched Fox News, or used his laptop and the hospital's wireless Internet to stay current on right-wing websites. Before I met Burt for the first time, he had Googled me and had me tagged as a public radio–listening, latte-sipping, left-leaning liberal (all true). And he was eager for a fight.

"But his persona was ninety percent bravado. To me—or anyone skilled at reading people—Burt was an open book. Within about five minutes of meeting him, it was evident that he thoroughly enjoyed people and valued friendships. He just loved arguing, particularly about politics. He wanted my help and our team's help, but I soon learned that we would have to deliver it on his terms.

"So political jousting became the currency of our daily visits. On most days, after my usual questions about his pain, how he slept, whether he had any appetite, and his bowels, he preferred to argue and advance his far-right political viewpoint. Through it all, Burt and I became friends. We could have serious conversations when we needed to—sometimes tender discussions about things that kept him awake some nights, things he regretted, including some that he had never told anyone else. According to the nurses on 1 West, who all knew Burt well, I also became a tonic for his anxieties and not-uncommon irritability.

"On one occasion, while in the hospital for a six-week stretch, Burt developed a serious infection—actually two infections, one bacterial and the other fungal—and was receiving high doses of potent antibiotics. Despite IV fluids and red blood cell transfusions whenever he became too anemic, the hematologists were having trouble keeping his blood pressure from falling. There was growing concern that he might need vasopressor medications, which would, in turn, require his being transferred to the ICU.

"When I visited he felt weak and had no appetite whatsoever, but said he was not in pain and did not otherwise feel ill. I noted to myself that he looked better than his 'labs,' or current blood counts, or the array of active medical problems in his chart. I felt hopeful he would once again pull through.

"The next morning I brought Burt something that I told him would help his recovery.

"On the wall of his room, directly in front of his bed, I taped an eight-by-eleven sheet of white paper on which I had printed in inch-high bold type: IN CASE OF LOW BLOOD PRESSURE, LIFT THIS PAGE. I explained that whenever his blood pressure got too low, I had instructed the nurses to lift and tape the cover sheet up. And I demon-strated, lifting the cover to reveal a color photo that I had copied from the Web and printed at home. It was of liberal cable TV talk show host Keith Olbermann, who stood with a large American flag behind him."

I told the class, "Burt rose up as if stung by a bee. 'I hate that sonofa-bitch!' he blurted out.

"'I think it's working!' I said. 'I bet your blood pressure is up by twenty points,' and I puffed out my chest and strutted around the room with mock therapeutic pride. That did it, the angry veneer collapsed, and Burt erupted in howls of laughter. Just then a nurse came in to see what the ruckus was about. Burt told her to report me to the authorities for abuse.

"We had a good laugh and I stayed for a while to allow him time to give me the right-wing news of the day, but (mercifully) my pager went off and I excused myself, saying I'd see him tomorrow.

"On rounds the following day, when I arrived at the counter of the charting station nearest his room, the nurses and aides were talking about the sign I had put up. They reported that Burt complains about it to everyone who visits—staff, family, and friends alike—but, they laughed, he hasn't taken it down."

The mood in the auditorium was lively. I only saw a couple of students

who seemed aloof or otherwise engaged. In body language and murmur-
ing, most evinced that blend of seriousness, perplexity, irony, and humor
that characterize true immersion in tough subjects. Pedagogic bliss.

I checked my watch again and decided to go further still.

"You have put up with me so far, but I suspect I may lose some of you
with what I am about to say about my approach to doctoring. I want to
let you in on my deepest therapeutic secret. I *imagine* my patients *well.*"

I assumed that this would sound flaky to at least a few students. As
faculty, we have been filling their minds with facts and the structure
and function of organs, cells, proteins, and genes, and I am talking about
imagination? Although it might sound "woo-woo" or New Agey to some
students, an informed imagination is a doctor's most powerful therapeutic tool. This applies to both physical and nonphysical realms of health.

"Imagining a person well suggests a route to an achievable destina-
tion. Particularly for patients who cannot be cured, this provides me
with a direction for counseling of seriously ill individuals and their
families. In fact, unless I am able to imagine a patient becoming 'well,'
it is unlikely I will be able to help the person find his or her own way to
well-being."

I explained that the ability to use one's imagination as a therapeutic
tool is a skill that they can develop and refine over the years of training
and practice ahead. At the beginning of clinical training it may be difficult for a medical student to envision "imagining a patient well" while
he or she is trying to remember which laboratory test or type of scan
to order, or which medication to use for a specific condition. I used the
analogy of an apprentice sculptor who is just learning to use the variety
of chisels, rasps, and mallets and must concentrate to avoid ruining a
piece of marble, contrasting the apprentice to a master sculptor who can
imagine the polished masterpiece within the uncut stone.

"In caring for people with far advanced illness, master physicians use
imagination in two tangible, directed ways. The first is in taking a history,
by listening carefully and trying to understand the perspective of the

patient. One person cannot fully know the intimate experience of another. That is why saying, 'I know what you're going through' can sound callous to a patient. However, if a physician has taken the time and invested the emotional energy to do so, she can say, 'I can only imagine how hard this must be for you,' in a way that conveys genuine empathy. Doctors can use their receptive imagination to listen to a patient's story as if they were the speaker and try to see the world through a patient's eyes.

"Once aligned with the personal perspective of a patient, a doctor's creative imagination is invaluable in counseling. I might ask a person to imagine the time ahead as part of an ongoing life story. 'Given what we know of the hero or heroine of this story, how might you hope for the story to unfold in the remaining chapters?'"

I explained that a physician's imagination can be a wellspring of people's hope.

"Hope is defined as 'a desire for some good, accompanied with at least a slight expectation of obtaining it, or a belief that it is obtainable.' Doctors can help people identify meaningful things they can still accomplish or achieve—and then work with them on a plan to do so."

I looked around the room. I had lost a few students' attention, but most were still with me.

"You have probably heard the nostrum, 'It is not what we do, but how *we are* that matters.' The exact words used in counseling a patient matter less than the doctor's confidence and ability to be fully present. A calm voice, unhurried pace, and willingness to listen can allay a person's fears. Perhaps on some level a patient feels, 'The doctor is not overwhelmed, so I must be all right.' Conversely, if a doctor is too uncomfortable to listen to a patient's concerns or too upset by the thought that a beloved patient may be dying, the doctor's own fears and anxiety can be contagious. We can be highly therapeutic simply by showing up, leaning forward, and listening attentively."

A student who hadn't said a word during the class, but had been leaning forward and clearly attentive throughout the afternoon, now raised her hand. She said, "I once heard a professor say that every doctor develops his or her own style of interacting with patients. How would you describe your style?"

I had never been asked that question. I had to think for a moment. My mind flipped through faces of patients I had cared for and counseled, and landed on Joyce.

"To be honest, in addition to using imagination in the way I just described, if I have a 'style,' I think it involves kibitzing."

I explained that gently kidding with and even lovingly teasing a patient enables me to gain a good sense of their quality of life, the state of their personhood. "I don't recommend this approach to everyone, but it works for me. Let me tell you about Joyce.

"Joyce was seventy-eight years old and looked as if she had spent most of those years out of doors. The wind had etched wizened lines around her expressive eyes and the sun had stretched her mouth into a permanent smile. Her daughter, Paula, and friends described Joyce as 'spry,' an indication of the feisty determination with which this sinewy Vermonter had lived. When her husband was seriously injured while felling a tree two days before his thirty-eighth birthday, becoming physically disabled and unemployed, Joyce held down a full-time bookkeeping job while also doing most of the chores on the small dairy farm the couple owned in northern Vermont.

"I had come to know Joyce over the better part of a year as our palliative care team helped her cope with the effects of chronic lymphoma. We were readily able to treat her pain, but she was gradually becoming weaker. Eventually the lymphoma was destined to claim Joyce's life. But not for a while. Hospitalized three days earlier with a chest cold that had become pneumonia, she had rapidly improved with IV antibiotics and was nearly ready for discharge. She was getting physically stronger every day, but on the day I visited she was still far too weak to take care of herself. Her spirits were at an all-time low.

"Joyce usually bantered with me. At our first visit, she had asked me about my 'accent' and where I'd grown up and since then often teased me about being from New Jersey. She loved *The Sopranos*, the TV show about Mafia families in New Jersey, and wanted to know if I was 'connected.' That afternoon, however, her mood was somber. We talked about her health and I said that it was probably no longer safe for her to be at home alone.

"I knew Joyce's family and was aware that her daughter, Paula, and eldest granddaughter, Ashley, along with Ashley's husband, Jarod, had repeatedly asked Joyce to live with them in southern Vermont. Joyce consistently resisted.

"'Paula's a patent attorney—and good at it—makes a very good living. But she is divorced, has three girls, one still in high school, and Ashley's pregnant. Don't get me wrong, Ira.' (We were on a first-name basis.) *'I love those kids like flowers love the rain,'* she added loudly. 'But Paula has her own problems. Bad relationships with a series of men— she picks real losers—and has never really found herself.' She gave me an if-ya-know-what-I-mean look. I nodded, indicating I was following the conversation. 'She's seeing a high-priced shrink in Albany. Two hundred dollars an hour'—Joyce rolled her eyes—'twice a week!'

"'I just want to stay in my own home—as long as I possibly can,' she said. Sitting in the recliner chair in her hospital room, Joyce confided in me, 'I really worry about becoming a burden to my family.'"

"I hoped gentle humor would get a rise out of her. 'You needn't worry, Joyce,' I said. 'I assure you, you already are.'"

"She chuckled and smiled wryly. 'Oh, thanks a lot. That makes me feel MUCH better.' A sparkle returned to her eyes.

"I explained that her family already owned her illness. 'How could it be otherwise? Your daughter and her children love you, and it's natural for them to worry about you. Do you really think it is easier on them with you so far away, living by yourself? The truth is, what they probably need most for their own peace of mind is to take care of you.'"

"She listened thoughtfully. 'Joyce,' I continued, 'didn't you tell me you had cared for both of your parents during the last part of their lives?'"

"'Yes.' She nodded.

"'And you cared for your husband for nearly ten years, including the months before his death. Was that important for you to do?'

"Nothing I said or asked that afternoon visibly moved Joyce as much as that question.

"'Yes, it was really important.' She nodded again.

"'When Paula was born, she required endless hours of care and, I'll bet, kept you up nights. Wasn't that a wee bit of a burden?' She kept my gaze but wasn't going to concede the point. 'Of course, she was a baby, for Christsakes!'

"'And when your husband was injured and you became the bread-winner for your family, as well as tending the farm, all the while caring for him—wasn't his condition and need for help a burden?'

"'Never for me!' she shot back.

"'How about for him? Did he ever express feeling that he was a bur-den on you and your family?' She looked down and, after a moment, nodded as if in a conversation with herself.

"'Yes, he did,' she said thoughtfully. 'For me, it just wasn't even a question. I loved him and did what I had to do.'

"'Joyce, my sense is that you have just described how Paula and your grandchildren feel now. You are their mother and grandmother, and they want to care for you. The fact is, they *need* to care for you, for their own emotional well-being. Their worse fear is having you die alone, maybe even on the floor of your farmhouse, with them miles away, unable to help.

"'Like it or not,' I continued, 'you and your family are in this together. Their lives are already disrupted by your illness. You can't fix that; you can only make the best of the situation. Consider that just possibly the best thing you can do for your family is to let them take care of you. They may need to pamper you to express their love for you.'

"I paused, before adding, 'And there are still lots of things you can do for your family that no one else can do.'

"'Like what?' she asked with a theatrical expression, her head tilted, one brow raised in doubt, the other eye squinted against potential evil. Apparently, she'd been warned about shysters from Jersey.

"'Well, for one thing you might consider telling your daughter that you are proud of being her mother. No one else on the planet can give her that gift.'

"At that point the theatrics evaporated and she abruptly began to tear up. I moved the box of tissues from her bedside table to the tray stand next to her recliner chair. Otherwise I was quiet, simply present, consciously creating a space in her hospital room in which she could do what she needed to do.

"After a few wordless moments, Joyce began to giggle. Curiosity got the best of me and I asked her what she was laughing about. Through her tears she said, 'That's what my daughter needs, Ira. She doesn't need that shrink! She needs *me*, her mother, to tell her I love her and that I'm proud of her!'

"We laughed together, agreeing that if all parents would take the time—and spend the emotional energy required—to tell each of our children how much we love them and how proud we are to be their mother or father, we might put a generation of psychotherapists out of business.

"'Another easy thing you might do is tell your stories. Maybe your daughter knows the details of your life, but do your grandchildren? Have they heard the history of where you grew up, about your brothers and sisters—their great-aunts and -uncles—when they were kids, and who your best friends were? Can they even imagine what your school was like, or your first job? Do they know the story of you and your husband meeting and falling in love?

"'You get my point. These are your stories, but in a sense, they are theirs, too. Our No One Alone volunteers often help people record their stories, usually just with a microphone, sometimes with the help of a family photo album. If you were to do it, I'd bet a lot that one day the child that Ashley is carrying will listen to those stories and hear your voice.'

"'Boy, you're good! You could probably sell snow to the Eskimos.'" She shook her head and smiled. I noted to myself that her remark changed the subject. Teasing me allowed her to avoid agreeing to anything.

"Still, something began to shift within Joyce that day. I telephoned her a couple of weeks after she left the hospital just to hear how she was doing. She said, 'As well as you could expect, I guess.' The friendly sarcasm in her voice let me know she was glad I called.

"She hadn't moved, but it was no longer out of the question. She allowed more paid help into her home. One granddaughter was now staying with her on weekends. And she said she'd taken my advice and begun recording some of her stories with the help of a hospice volunteer.

"I asked her whether it was hard for her to accept help from her daughter and granddaughters.

"'I don't like it,' she said, adding, 'but I guess that's life.'

I asked the students to notice how I had built on the rapport I had established with Joyce—and employed imagination in counseling her.

"This is the sort of counseling that mostly requires a bit of time and the will to listen. This therapy is safe and nontoxic, and not esoteric. Even medical students can do it!"

That brought open laughter. At this point the auditorium felt like a living room. People were relaxed and our time was drawing to a close.

A student raised her hand and then said she had a serious question. "You clearly get close to your patients. What is the cost of caring to you? How do you deal with your feelings, especially during busy days?"

"Well, there are plenty of days that I feel drained. I am often glad for the evenings and the weekends I am not on call, and for vacations. Luckily I have a wife and children who love me, and a full personal life that balances the stresses and sorrows that I experience as a doctor. Sleep, exercise, meditation, good food, and humor all help a lot.

"Be wary of the notion that we doctors are like glasses that are either full or empty. In this view our emotional tanks are inevitably drained by our jobs. This assumption disserves us. In my practice, I am more often filled up by my relationships with patients, including those who are dying. After more than thirty years of practice, I often walk out of the hospital at night feeling struck with how lucky I am to do what I do. Sometimes, I feel that way even when someone I have cared a lot about dies."

As the class ended, I reminded the students to complete an evaluation form and said again that I hoped they would choose this topic for next year's ICE class.

Gathering my papers and walking from the auditorium, my thoughts went back to the student's last question about the emotional toll this work sometimes exacts from me. My thoughts went to a young patient whose hard life and illness affected me deeply and I remembered the day that Sharon died.

7.

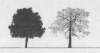

The Busy Day
That Sharon Died

The clock on my bedside table read 4:42 a.m. I had awakened from a bad dream. I was drenched in sweat and vividly recalled crawling my way to the surface from a dark, stifling dreamscape cave.

As I lay without stirring in my bed, I could still see that place with dank walls and a scrawny gray creature that reminded me of Gollum from *Lord of the Rings*. It was vaguely threatening, but also hurt and needy. It crouched, staring up at me from a small pool of water it was protecting. I recognized that the being represented Sharon, a seventeen-year-old patient who suffered from cystic fibrosis, a congenital disease that clogs airways and eventually destroys the architecture of the lungs. Sharon was known as the "Princess of Darkness" of our pediatric ward. She was frequently hospitalized—enough to have a favorite room and be cranky if she didn't get it.

Sharon was dying, and it didn't take an analyst to recognize the dream as my psyche wrestling with my sadness and almost nauseating sense of unfairness. She was a good kid who had done nothing wrong!

I sometimes wake thinking about the patients I will see that day and suspecting that one or another will die. This morning, I awoke feeling in my gut that it would be the day that Sharon died.

My wife, Yvonne, stirred but fell back to sleep as I padded into the bathroom.

"If looks could kill, there'd be a pile of dead doctors and nurses at her door," Dr. Jorge Ruiz told me on the day he invited me to become involved in Sharon's care. His facial expression said, "This is not going to be easy."

It had been more than two years ago that Jorge, her pulmonary specialist, asked me to help alleviate Sharon's pain and GI (gastrointestinal) symptoms. He also asked me to help her and her mother adjust to what Jorge called "her unrelenting decline." He didn't need to say, "and her coming death." The tone of his voice and doleful eyes said enough.

It was mid-afternoon when I first went to see her, yet Sharon's room was dim. I knocked on her door. No response. A curtain was drawn around her bed. Over the years, I have learned that, in many ways, patients open themselves and their stories to me as a physician, but that I must be willing and able to read them.

"Hello? I am Dr. Byock," I said, poking my head into her room. "May I come in?"

I waited at the threshold and then waited some more. "I guess," an adolescent voice finally responded.

I pulled aside the curtains to reveal an empty, unmade bed with an IV pole on its far side, festooned with bags of saline and medications. The settings of patients' hospital rooms often tell a lot about the people within—their personalities, moods, interests, and values; their families (often people tape or pin pictures to the bulletin board or walls); their styles. These walls were bare. And where was Sharon?

"Hellooo?" I said again.

"I'm over here." I peered over the bed's edge. An untouched lunch tray sat atop teen magazines on the bedside table, next to *The Illustrated*

Encyclopedia of North American Reptiles and Amphibians. Sharon sat cross-legged on the floor, amid a sprawl of clothes that seemed to have spilled from the open rolling suitcase not far away. She was working on a bead necklace in a design that resembled intricate Moroccan latticework. She did not look up, and I could not see her face, which was hidden by straight, shoulder-length light brown hair, parted in the middle.

Her fingertips were swollen like the ends of Q-tips, one of the common signs, or stigmata, of chronic lung disease. Low levels of oxygen at the tips of fingers and toes of people with CF, emphysema, or other respiratory disease can cause blood vessels and soft tissues to hypertrophy, rounding the normally concave junction of the cuticles and nails.

She was wearing a well-worn black sweatshirt. Chipped black nail polish adorned all digits but her left pinky on which the oxygen saturation sensor was taped. Her slender hands vibrated in a fine tremor, impressing me with the patience and concentration it must have required to string those tiny beads.

"I'm Dr. Byock," I repeated. "I work with something called the Palliative Care Service."

"I know who you are. You're Dr. Death," she said. Without missing a beat, she speared a few more beads with the long needle. It's common for people to assume that palliative care has something to do with dying, but "Dr. Death" is the nickname most often used to refer to suicide doctor Jack Kevorkian. I wanted to distance myself as far as possible from that association.

I looked down at Sharon's oily, uncombed, straight head of hair. I could see only her nose, which poked through the brown to nearly blond strands of hair as if peeking through a curtain of strings.

People sometimes wonder if doctors can see through them—metaphorically, of course. Before going to medical school, I used to wonder how much experienced physicians could tell about me, or anyone, just by looking. The truth is: quite a lot. It is the inevitable result of training and experience.

Doctors are trained to be observant. We tend to pay attention to things like the condition of a person's hands: Are they rough or soft? Do they have calluses, nicotine-stained fingers, carefully filed or chewed nails? Similarly, we take note of a person's teeth and skin, the lines in his or her face. And then there is people's grooming, or lack thereof, and the style of their hair and clothes: what they chose or had to wear to the doctor's office.

Such things can tell us a lot about a person's habits and also about their life in general. Through the eyes of an experienced physician, a person's history is revealed—not the specifics, of course, as we are not mind readers—but the tenor of a person's life, the general extent of strain, and the cumulative toll experience has taken. People's expressions and mannerisms, their posture and gaze, whether they fidget or are calmly posed—all contribute to a general impression of their inner state.

"Well, actually, I like to think what I do is about *living*," I replied. "Our team focuses on people's comfort and quality of life, and helps people who are dealing with difficult courses of treatment." I paused, giving her a chance to respond. She didn't.

"You don't have to be dying for us to help," I continued. "You just have to be seriously ill. I understand that, unfortunately, you are pretty ill."

"Yu-up," she said with a sarcastic inflection, as if she were saying, *"DUH-uuh."*

I felt we were fencing, and I decided to thrust. "But tell me, are you dying?"

"Yeah, I know I'm going to die."

I noted to myself that saying "I'm going to die" is not the same as saying "I'm dying." I asked Sharon what it meant to her to know that she was going to die.

"Nothing," she said. "When you've been told three hundred times that you are going to die, who cares? Unless I can get a transplant..." she added softly. That caveat apparently didn't diminish her apathy, because she spoke louder in asking, "So what?"

She barely moved her shoulders, in a half shrug, a kind of resigned gesture meant to say, "My life is lousy. Tell me something I don't know."

I followed Sharon's lead in downplaying the subject of a lung transplant. In fact, I wondered how realistic a lung transplant was for Sharon and if she knew what she'd be getting into. Doctors often refer to receiving a transplant as exchanging one serious illness for another. A transplanted lung can extend a patient's life by an average of five years—given the alternative, that's a lot—but they can be arduous and uncomfortable years. Then again, the bell survival curve around the five-year midpoint is wide, meaning that a few people live many years longer, while others die shortly after receiving their new lung.

I decided to stay focused on what made her tick. "You know, I am here because Dr. Ruiz and a few of the nurses think you are depressed. They are worried about you and asked our team to see if we could help. Do you think you are depressed?"

"I suppose. Why wouldn't I be? My life is shit," she said. And just then she looked up, her hair falling to the sides of her face as she cocked her head, and met my eyes full on. It was the slightest of motions, yet I had the distinct impression that she had been saving the move for effect. Sharon's narrow face, still that of a pretty young girl, had the gaunt look of an old woman. The absence of natural subcutaneous fat around her nose and orbital ridges set her dark brown eyes deep within their sockets, accentuating dark crescents under her eyes. Looking at Sharon was like staring back at a subject in a photojournalist's series of war-torn refugees or Dorothea Lange's historical photos from the Dust Bowl. She was malnourished. Her deprivation was not from lack of food but from the physiologic inability to absorb the nutrients she ate.

She knew the effect her appearance had on strangers. I'm sure she had seen people flinch at the sight of her and look away. I understood why "breaks my heart" was a phrase often spoken by the pediatric nurses when they talked about Sharon.

———————

THAT WAS TWO years earlier. Last night I had set my alarm for 5:15 and, now that I was awake, decided to start the day. Shaking off my dream and early-morning reverie, I quickly shaved and showered. From the bathroom window I saw that fresh snow had fallen overnight and blown into a two-foot drift against our garage door. I dressed and scanned from my laptop the dozen or so e-mails that had arrived overnight. Most were junk mail, notices, or newsletters, but two were serious and time sensitive. Whenever possible, I adopt a "touch it once" strategy with correspondence, particularly during weeks when I am the attending physician for our inpatient consultation team. It was just the second day of my seven-day stretch. Days would be long through next weekend, and e-mails—as well as projects and committee work that required my attention—could easily pile up. The more tasks I could touch once and complete, the better.

Each took a few minutes to read and respond to. I put my computer into pause mode. I knew I was running a few minutes late. Nevertheless, I took time to meditate.

Long ago, I realized that sitting in meditation was the single most important thing I could do to prepare for each day. The twenty minutes I invest pay off by enabling me to be more fully present and in the moment as I see patients and families who are in dizzying, deeply distressing situations. Whenever I skip meditation, sometime during the course of the day I notice that I need to expend extra effort to maintain my equilibrium as events and emotions threaten to push or pull me off center.

During my meditation this morning, images of the creature from my dream kept arising. There she was, squatting on the cluttered floor of her room, peering up at me. Snippets from the past twenty-six months ran across my mind's eye—a series of grayscale snapshots of Sharon sitting against monochrome floors, walls, and privacy drapes.

Sharon had been frequently hospitalized, usually for one to three weeks at a time, during the period since I met her. During her times in the hospital we had forged a doctor-patient relationship that gradually became a doctor-patient friendship. I would usually stop by to see her at the end of my hospital day, my last task before heading home. Sometimes I would bring her a bottle of sugarless flavored water from the gift shop, one of the only "treats" she was officially allowed.

Sharon was tough and often infuriated nurses, phlebotomists, respiratory therapists, and radiology techs. But she was also transparent. Her crankiness was clearly behavioral armor worn by a frightened child. She was vulnerable but not defenseless. When it came to treatments, medications, and her diet, there were things she was willing to do and things she refused. She would split the staff, currying favor from some while giving the cold shoulder to others. Sharon distinguished between those who "understood" her (that is, cut her some slack) whom she allowed to work with her, and those she didn't like and would not talk to. Sometimes she would simply pretend to do what Dr. Ruiz or the pediatric residents and nurses asked, or would sneak something forbidden, like a sugary treat— a potential catastrophe for her fluctuating blood sugar levels.

Late one afternoon, during my second visit, it was pretty obvious that Sharon was feeling low. I was still trying to establish some rapport. Although I could think of any number of reasons why Sharon might be depressed, I wanted to know which ones gnawed at her most.

"I wonder," I began, "if you couldn't change having CF, but could change something else, can you imagine anything that would make your life more worth living?"

"Boobs!" she said, without hesitation.

Touché! I thought. We were fencing again and I was parrying with a pro. "Well," I chuckled aloud, "sounds like an entirely reasonable thing for someone your age to want." I was a family doctor earlier in my career, and am the father of two now adult daughters. Breasts are a normal thing for an adolescent girl to want. Menarche typically occurs when girls are between eleven and thirteen years old, but at fifteen, Sharon had not yet had a period. She had breast buds noted on a recent physical examination by a pediatric resident—small nodules of early breast tissue under her nipples—but to her, they were just another reminder that she was not yet a woman. She said she felt abnormal and ugly. I said that her thinness was probably keeping her from developing breasts and, in an attempt to offer a nonpathologic context to the problem, reflected that many young ballerinas and gymnasts are late in developing breasts, as well as starting their periods.

"Yup," she nodded, this time without irony. I was reinforcing what she already understood about the biology of her condition. I hoped I was also earning some professional credibility in her eyes.

It was hard to know. Sharon went on speaking openly about her sexual development, yet she did so without emotion, somehow distant from her body. She said "I" as though referring to someone in the third person.

"I know I need to gain weight in order to grow breasts, but I don't know if I can," she said. The rising tone of her voice told me she still had hopes. She'd allowed me to see what really mattered. Seeds of trust had been planted.

"If growing breasts is high on your priority list for improving your quality of life, then we will do whatever we can to help you gain the weight you need," I told her before I left.

Now, two years later, Sharon was seventeen and quickly approaching the ledge of life. As I continued to meditate, that knowledge loomed in my consciousness like a storm cloud. Long ago, I had come to accept that Sharon's dark hospital room was for her a safe cocoon, so I wondered why the cave in my dream felt foreboding. I suspected that below the level of my usual awareness, I was wrestling with my awareness that Sharon could very well die today.

I rose from my cushion. I walked to the kitchen, poured a cup of coffee, tied my tie, and dressed for the cold. As the garage door flipped open, I started the car and then grabbed the snow shovel leaning against the garage wall. Midwinter mornings in the mountains of New Hampshire can be brutally cold. It was 10 degrees Fahrenheit, with gusting wind. Nonetheless, after I had heaved away the worst of the drift, I took a moment to appreciate the starry sky. It was as much of nature as I would see that day. My weeks as attending physician on our inpatient service are particularly intense: I would not leave the hospital until 6:30 or 7:00 p.m., hours after the sun had set again.

To fulfill my mission as a palliative care doctor to protect patients' comfort and well-being, I also have to improve care systems. That's why I was headed to the 6:45 a.m. Tumor Board on this cold Tuesday morning. Medical, surgical, and radiation oncologists use this weekly meeting to discuss new cancer cases. My presence tends to expand the discussions, encouraging them to consider the impact of potential treatments on each patient's quality of life.

Thankfully, I-89, my route to the hospital in Lebanon, had been plowed and well sanded. I switched on NPR and caught the last of the bottom-of-the-hour headlines. But my thoughts went back to Sharon and I turned the radio off.

A lot had happened since that first meeting with Sharon. She was admitted to CHaD—the Children's Hospital at Dartmouth—every few months, and more recently almost every month. Usually she came in because of a chest infection that started with a low-grade fever, mild shortness of breath, and achy "respirophasic" right chest pain that hurt whenever she took a deep breath or coughed, and kept getting worse despite oral antibiotics. A few times it was because her blood sugars were dangerously high—in the mid-400s, with normal being about 100—and could not be controlled as an outpatient.

None of this was new to her. It was just the latest phase of the only life she had ever known.

Shortly after birth, Sharon had been diagnosed with an intestinal blockage. Tests revealed elevated chloride in her sweat that led to the diagnosis of cystic fibrosis. CF, as it's called, affects roughly thirty thousand Americans. It's a deadly disease to have (although recent advances in genetics, proteomics, and drug development are raising hopes for dramatically effective new treatments and making it possible to even imagine a cure). CF increases the viscosity of secretions—think mucus—particularly in the respiratory tract, causing chronic sinusitis and bronchitis, and gradually destroying the delicate grapelike clusters of air sacks, the alveoli, which provide the surface area for exchanging oxygen and carbon dioxide between our lungs and bloodstream.

Normally, the mucus in our sinuses, bronchi, and lungs is liquid, the consistency of warm honey. People affected by CF have mucus with the consistency of caramel. This impedes the fine hairlike cilia that rhythmically beat, usually sweeping mucus upward and outward, continually cleansing our lower airways.

CF is best known as a respiratory disease, but it is also a disease of the gut and endocrine system, and it can cause cirrhosis of the liver.

Sharon had it all. In addition to a daily regimen of twelve different pills, she inhaled foul detergent-like mists and antibiotic sprays every few hours to loosen her clotted secretions. For fifteen minutes, three times a day, she also endured "cupping and clapping" treatments—a therapist or her mom beating on her chest—or, when they were not available, she was strapped into a special vibration vest, which resembles a medieval torture jacket with only the ancient sharp iron spikes replaced by rows of stiff tubes that deliver alternating sharp bursts of compressed air from a pump to literally shake the spit out of her. She needed insulin injections twice a day, and as often as every four hours if her blood glucose tested high. She was prone to infections and slow to heal. Diabetes put her at risk for premature aging of the small arteries leading to her kidneys, and eye and heart problems, although, as Sharon was acutely aware, she was unlikely to live long enough to suffer those complications.

During my first handful of visits, I had focused mostly on building trust and a "therapeutic relationship." I teach students, residents, and fellows that a physician's genuine concern and positive regard for the person can engender comfort and confidence. Cynics who dismiss this as a placebo effect miss its significance. Therapeutic rapport is legitimate; it's an invaluable clinical resource and an attribute of being a "real doctor." Its effect can be more powerful than Valium. Indeed, the Valium-like benzodiazepine class of drugs—Ativan, Xanax, Serax, Librium, and Klonopin, to name a few—give people a "mother's at home" sense of well-being. Seasoned doctors know that their presence and caring can be every bit as effective.

During another visit early in our relationship, I asked Sharon what else might be on her fantasy wish list, reminding her that I was not a genie and was asking as a way of getting to know her better as a person. She wished for a Tempur-Pedic mattress, a pet dog, a nose job, interest from boys, and to learn ballet. She adored animals: her secret wish was to become a veterinarian when she grew up. She said "when" with an inflection that let me know she meant "if." She had a pet lizard, Gizmo, but was worried that she would have to give him away because no one gave him attention during her frequent hospitalizations.

Sharon's family lived near Manchester, New Hampshire, an hour and a quarter's drive south of our hospital. They had plenty of challenges. There was a lot of love among them and never a hint of malice, but they were often in turmoil. Sharon's parents had divorced when she was eight. She was fourteen when her mother, Stephanie, remarried; just three months later, her stepfather, Bill, suffered a stroke that paralyzed his left arm and leg, rendering him unable to work. Money had been tight before his illness, and now it was a constant worry. They were forced to move to a smaller apartment. Her limited mobility and the family's small quarters felt stifling to Sharon, particularly during the long, cold New England winters. Even trips in the car were limited. When she was in the hospital, the high price of gas limited her family to visiting only on weekends.

Three years ago our team created a special patient amenities fund to give people in situations like Stephanie and Bill's a few prepaid "gas cards" to defray some of the costs of their visits. We also contributed $50 to a fund that CHaD nurses created to purchase a hypoallergenic hairless cat for Sharon, a truly grotesque-looking creature that she cherished and named Chloe. As luck would have it Chloe promptly contracted a feline virus, had to have an infected eye removed, and died just six months after Sharon first held the creature in her arms—a series of events that only seemed to confirm Sharon's brooding belief that she was cursed. But Sharon accepted Chloe's death with characteristic stoicism. It was simply par for the course.

Sometimes on a Saturday when Sharon was in the hospital and my schedule permitted, I arranged for a "pass" that enabled her to leave the premises. I'd take her to a pet store for an hour or so. She was elated, pointing out every variety of dog, rabbit, snake, and spider. She transformed from the terror of the ward to a normal kid, developmentally younger than her midteen years, brimming with the energy of youth. If her stomach was up to it, we would stop for a lunch of her favorite nonhospital food: tuna melts, and a special off-diet treat, ice cream.

Through our innumerable appointments and conversations, Sharon, Stephanie, and I gradually built a doctor-patient-parent relationship that allowed for an easy, ongoing to-and-fro of information and ideas. Even when Sharon was not in the hospital, I heard from her mother regularly, usually by e-mail and occasionally by phone. Stephanie's e-mails were typically short, usually letting me know about a minor change in Sharon's bowel symptoms or her difficulty getting a medication approved by Medicaid. Sometimes she would send me an e-mail just to brag that Sharon had completed a dance class and hung her certificate on her bedroom wall, or had done unexpectedly well on a standardized test at school. If more than a week or two went by without an update, I would check her chart or call and check in.

During a CHaD care planning meeting I attended, one of the social workers wondered aloud whether the special attention some of us gave

Sharon was appropriate. By "appropriate," she meant ethical. Why her and not other patients? Weren't we crossing a sacrosanct professional boundary between doctor or nurse and patient?

I took the matter seriously, but not from lack of confidence in the propriety of my actions. I considered the concern a teachable moment. Our team used our regular weekly education meetings to discuss these issues. Professional boundaries serve to protect vulnerable patients from manipulative doctors. But clear professional boundaries also free physicians and patients to be authentic with one another. We had lively discussions and came to the conclusion that befriending people who happen to be our patients is not a transgression. Whenever possible, we decided, we *should* pamper our patients. Laura Rollano said it best: "Sometimes it's okay to take a kid to a pet store."

Far from representing a violation of professional boundaries, I felt it was a privilege to help Sharon. I made her life a little better in simple ways, by truly *caring for her*. It would have been inauthentic to suppress the impulse to do so, which after all is at the fundamental core of medicine. I had earned the privilege by showing up, again and again, and being present during the lowest times in her struggle to live in the face of relentless disease.

All the efforts of her doctors, nurses, pharmacists, nutritionists, and respiratory therapists could not keep Sharon from gradually, inexorably becoming sicker. We adjusted her pain medications, using a low dose of long-acting morphine three times a day so that she would not have to ask for every dose. The nurses could also give her quick-acting morphine for breakthrough pain. With this medication, Sharon was more comfortable and considerably less cranky. She was also more willing to wear her percussion jacket.

Despite Sharon's considerable efforts to eat, her nutrition got worse rather than better, and her prospects of developing breasts dimmed. Suspecting that her cramping and diarrhea were partly due to acquired lactose intolerance, I tried but failed to convince her to use Lactaid milk and ice cream. She scrunched her face and insisted it wouldn't taste good. After several months, Stephanie and Sharon decided on surgery to place a PEG tube through her abdominal wall into her stomach. The liquid nutrients (you couldn't call them "food" by any stretch of the imagination) caused painful cramping in her intestines and gave her even more diarrhea.

As summer became fall, she grew thinner and more skeletal and wizened in appearance. Working on beads or schoolwork, she often curled herself up in positions that resembled the poses of ascetic yogis. She would "cocoon" in her hospital room, a common approach among teenagers for coping with the unpleasant realities of life.

Sharon kept the room dark and left strict instructions not to be disturbed as she slept through the mornings into the early afternoons. I came to see her cocooning as a futile attempt to magically emerge into a brighter and happier world. She desperately wanted a future, although she knew that she was destined to die before the transformation could occur. But she was still a warm, loving, and colorful teenage girl.

Sharon had recently been rejected from the lung transplant list at a hospital in Boston because of the extent of her liver disease and gastrointestinal malabsorption. Her chest pain had increased, and her abdominal cramps made even the brief periods between her respiratory treatments miserable. She frequently avoided respiratory treatments by pulling the blankets of her hospital bed over her head and refusing to budge. Whenever I visited now, I focused on doing whatever was possible to help her tolerate treatments and get stronger. Despite doing everything we could think of to make the best of this difficult predicament, Sharon and her mother had begun talking with each other, and to me, about stopping her treatments and accepting her dying.

Sharon missed her family and her friends from school and church, whom she rarely saw when she was at CHaD. She told me that she didn't want to spend the rest of her life in the hospital. "If I am not going to get better, what's the point?"

I PULLED onto the loop drive that encircles the Dartmouth-Hitchcock medical complex. I parked my car and stepped into the freezing wind. I pushed the electronic key fob with my gloved fingers to lock the car doors behind me and hurried toward the hospital. It was time to attend to the business at hand: tumor board from 6:45 a.m. to 7:45 a.m. and then our team's morning "huddle."

At our daily eight o'clock morning meeting, we discuss each of the patients on The List and plan the work of the day: how to manage various patients' symptoms, help them adjust to their illness and prognosis, and, always, assist them in navigating the complex maze of the health care system. Responsibility for chairing the meeting rotates. Today it was chaired by Karen Grocholski, our chaplain and spiritual services coordinator. Among the team members participating were: Annette Macy, another attending physician; Laura Rollano, social worker; two nurse practitioners; the triage nurse; the massage therapist; and the manager of our volunteer program. As director, I participate whether or not I am "on service," meaning that day's attending physician for the clinical team.

The "huddle" starts promptly at 8:00 a.m. We begin with a poem as a way of separating the events of our personal lives and the world from the work we come together to do as a team. This morning, Betty Priest, a nurse practitioner, read "To be of use" by Marge Piercy.

> *The people I love the best*
> *jump into work head first*
> *without dallying in the shallows*
> *and swim off with sure strokes almost out of sight.*
> *They seem to become natives of that element,*
> *the black sleek heads of seals*
> *bouncing like half submerged balls.*

I love people who harness themselves, an ox to a heavy cart,
who pull like water buffalo, with massive patience,
who strain in the mud and the muck to move things forward,
who do what has to be done, again and again.

I want to be with people who submerge
in the task, who go into the fields to harvest
and work in a row and pass the bags along,
who stand in the line and haul in their places,
who are not parlor generals and field deserters
but move in a common rhythm
when the food must come in or the fire be put out.

The work of the world is common as mud.
Botched, it smears the hands, crumbles to dust.
But the thing worth doing well done
has a shape that satisfies, clean and evident.
Greek amphoras for wine or oil,
Hopi vases that held corn, are put in museums
but you know they were made to be used.
The pitcher cries for water to carry
and a person for work that is real.

After the poem, the pace of the huddle quickens, as we have a lot to do in less than an hour. There were fifteen patients we were following in the hospital, and the outpatient clinic schedule was fairly full, with two nurse practitioners each scheduled to see eight patients.

First on our agenda was Deaths, the section on The List that contains the names of any of our patients who died during the past twenty-four hours. There are one to three deaths on a typical day. We meet most of the people we care for during turbulent times in their lives, and it feels important to us all to know how each story ends. It doesn't happen automatically. Many of our patients live in communities an hour or more away from the medical center and are cared for by their own doctors, community hospitals, nursing homes, and hospice programs in their own communities. Often no one thinks to notify the specialists they have seen at our medical center. So we have developed our own system of sending death notices any of us receive from colleagues to our secretaries, who also daily scan regional newspapers for obituaries. This allows us to make a follow-up call to each family of the patients we serve to learn how the person died and to assess how each family is doing in the immediate aftermath of their loved one's death.

After Deaths, we discussed the Outpatients Who Are In, a section compiled from scanning the electronic records for patients who have been admitted to the hospital overnight. This morning there were two— one was having radiosurgery, an outpatient procedure to treat a single metastatic brain tumor. He would only be at the medical center for about five hours and did not need to be seen by us. The other was Alex, a man with melanoma who was being admitted for swelling and pain in his left groin. We added him to the Inpatient section of The List and planned to see him on rounds.

Next were Outpatient Challenges, and in this context, I updated the team about Sharon's situation. It was just last Monday that she and her mother decided to go home and receive hospice care. I left for a conference in Chicago early the next morning, and although I had entered my notes in her medical chart and related the events to Helen Walek, the nurse practitioner I work with most closely on our inpatient service, I had not yet had a chance to discuss the transition and current plan of care at a morning huddle.

Helen and I had worked together for nearly six years and had come to know each other very well. At thirty-seven years of age, the mother of two, Helen had a peaches and cream complexion, warm smile, and an unwavering determination to take the best care possible of people in the worst of circumstances. Some days, I think Helen and I are a bit like partners on television cop shows. We know each other's style and can usually tell what the other is thinking or feeling about a clinical situation.

Helen is from the first generation of nurse practitioner specialists in palliative care. Upon graduating nursing school, she worked in a hospital in Cleveland for three years before taking a position as a home hospice nurse. She had a natural ability to soothe people in distress. She also discovered an interest in the science of medicine and enrolled in a master's program, becoming a nurse practitioner with the ability to diagnose and treat most clinical problems. Helen joined the team at Dartmouth-Hitchcock Medical Center the year before I was recruited.

At Dartmouth, nurse practitioners function as essential, respected members of clinical teams. On our team, the nurse practitioners perform consultations and care for patients in clinic, very much as I and the other physicians in our group do. Formally, the nurse practitioners rely on us for oversight and supervision. And they do. But informally, we collaborate and rely on one another.

I began reporting in matter-of-fact fashion: Sharon is at home, with her mother and stepfather there 24/7 and good support from their church and extended family, including people coming from out of town. She is receiving 7.5 milligrams of oral methadone twice a day, with 10 milligrams of high-concentration oral morphine solution as needed for breakthrough pain or breathlessness. A Hospice SOS Kit is also in the home, with injectable medications and supplies to control severe symptoms if needed.

When I finished, Helen said, "You know, Ira, I am going to be keeping my eyes on you." She looked around the large conference table—which is actually three folding tables placed together. The majority of our team was present for the morning huddle, in addition to Alison, a medical student, and Christopher, an internal medicine resident.

"We all get closer to some patients than to others. Sharon and you clearly have a special bond." Helen spoke in the formal tone someone uses when speaking up at a public forum. While her words were spoken to me with an "I'm just sayin'" attitude, they were intended for everyone in the room, including the two trainees.

The room was quiet. Helen turned and addressed the rest of the team. "As everyone here, except perhaps Alison and Christopher, knows, Ira has been the only one of us who Sharon will actually talk with. She has been polite to me but mostly declines to see anyone else. So this is not one of the usual situations in which we can share the burden. Last Thursday, while Ira was away, I got a call from Sharon's hospice nurse about her morphine dose. Alison and I read through some of his recent entries in her chart during her last admission when she had another exacerbation and a lot of pain. I want to read a few excerpts from the notes to give you all a sense of what's been going on."

She flipped through the electronic hospital records and read the narrative portion of the progress notes I had written:

PALLIATIVE CARE INPATIENT PROGRESS NOTE

Patient: Sharon Valero
DOB: 05/18/1989
PCP: Jorge Ruiz, M.D.
Consultant: Ira Byock, M.D.
Date: Friday, January 20, 2006

I visited Sharon in her room this afternoon before the weekend in follow-up to a long visit we had early last evening. She had just awakened from a nap, but was willing to talk.

She was alert, fully oriented. She has a frequent harsh, moist cough with tachypnea (at ~22/min) and use of accessory muscles. She spoke in full sentences. Affect mostly flat, becoming tearful at times. But she was friendly and, by the end of the visit, managed to smile.

She said she was feeling "okay," but admitted that her breathing is still "not great." When I asked how she was really doing, she said, "Sad." I gently probed, acknowledging her cat, Chloe's, recent death, but questioning whether there was more than that that was making her sad. She broke down in tears and talked about many aspects of her life that are hard. She wants to get out of the hospital but knows that she'll just be alone, all day every day, in her room when she's at home. Without her cat or another pet, she feels isolated and alone in her room. She also said, "I'll be home for a while and then I'll just get sick again and come back to the hospital."

She still really wants a transplant but knows it is a long shot and feels tired and isn't sure how long she can keep going.

I gently explored whether there would come a time when she might decide not to come back to the hospital. She said that she thinks about it pretty often, but that "I can't give up because of my mom. She wants me to keep fighting." I replied that I want her to get well, too, but reminded her that her mother had approved the idea of starting hospice care so that Sharon could get more of her care at home and that she would have the option of staying there through the end of her life, instead of coming back to the hospital, if and when she decided to do so.

I asked if she had spoken with Bob, her younger brother, recently. She said she hadn't called him and didn't want to impose on him. "He has his own problems," Sharon replied. I asked if she'd heard from her father. Yes, her father had recently invited her to travel next summer with him and his wife (Sharon's stepmother) to Europe. Sharon was delighted, but worries that she will not be well enough to go. I offered to call her father and explain her precarious medical situation and ask him to come visit. "No," she said, it would just frighten him and he doesn't do well with people on the phone. I then wondered aloud if, despite all her own problems, Sharon was protecting me (from talking with her father), her father from the news of how ill she was, and Bob, whom she loves and misses. Yes, she nodded, and acknowledged through her tears that she was protecting all of them—and her mother, too, from the knowledge of how ill she is and how bad she often feels.

I suggested that it was high time for her to allow those of us— professionals and her friends and family—who are not seriously ill and care about her to take care of her, pamper her, and make her comfortable. She was willing to consider allowing me to call her father.

She is looking forward to her mother visiting on Friday. She feels her pain is better controlled with the current dose of methadone (7.5mg oral twice a day).

Assess: I'm concerned about Sharon's physical condition; her lack of significant improvement, her general malaise, low-grade fevers, oxygen requirements.

Her depressed mood is an amalgam of depression and grief.

PLAN: I will continue to assist with supportive counseling and problem-solving whenever possible. Hospice care at home is available through Community Home Health and Hospice out of Nashua.

I hope to talk with Sharon's mother this weekend.

/ Ira Byock, M.D.

PALLIATIVE CARE INPATIENT PROGRESS NOTE

Patient: Sharon Valero
DOB: 05/18/89
PCP: Jorge Ruiz, M.D.
Consultant: Ira Byock, M.D.
Date: Monday, January 23, 2006

Following my last visit with Sharon, I asked the CHaD nurses to have her mother contact me by e-mail. Below is an e-mail I rec'd from Sharon's mother, Stephanie, from yesterday. Please see the Progress Note that follows.

Subject: Let's Talk
Date: January 22, 2006
From: Stephanie@NewHampshire.net

Ira,

I would very much like to talk with you about Sharon. We're both depressed, and although I don't think I show it around her, it's becoming increasingly difficult for her to hang on. She's told me she wants to give up and that all she wants to do is crawl inside a nice warm place and sleep forever.

If you get this message today, I'll be at home after church. If not, then I'll be at work tomorrow.

Thanks,
Stephanie

Stephanie contacted me on Sunday (01/22) and we subsequently spoke at length by phone.

She has come to the realization that Sharon is not getting better. Sharon told her that she is extremely tired and wants to give up. Stephanie is overwhelmed with sadness, but is also confident that it is the correct course of action. She said, "I feel like telling Dr. Ruiz not to bother with the transplant evaluation. Sharon just doesn't have it in her. I know that in my heart and soul." She added, "There is no joy in her anymore."

She wept as we talked. I asked her if she had any clarity re: where she would want Sharon to be cared for during this last phase of her life.

Stephanie has been in touch with a hospice intake coordinator at Community Home Health and Hospice in Nashua, which has a pediatric hospice team. The hospice program had deferred coming out to meet her b/c Sharon was readmitted. Last evening during our phone call I asked Stephanie to recontact them to say that I wanted the hospice to meet Stephanie and begin the admissions process, so that contingency plans could be put in place.

Stephanie sent an e-mail last evening, asking for my assistance in contacting Red Cross to facilitate a family medical leave from the military for her son, Eddie, to visit. Stephanie also gave me permission to contact her ex-husband and Sharon's father, Albert, to inform him of Sharon's condition and encourage him to visit.

Stephanie said that current neighbors of theirs, Sandy and Zeke Graber, had offered to help in any way they can and had prevailed upon Bill, Stephanie's husband, to allow them to get another cat for Sharon.

PLAN: I will contact hospice to re-activate the evaluation and admissions process.

I will contact Red Cross to begin the process of emergency family medical leave for Eddie.

I will try to call Sharon's father to apprise him of the situation and encourage a visit.

Our palliative care team is available to work with the peds team to facilitate transition to home hospice care if that continues to be the direction Sharon and her family decide to pursue—and to support Sharon, her mother and the peds team here in any way we can. (I will be away from the hospital on Tuesday through Friday this week.)

/ Ira Byock, M.D.

HELEN LOOKED up from her laptop. "Man, Ira, I have to tell you, I've got a lump in my throat."

I suddenly understood why, yesterday, Alison had asked why I chart in the way that I do. I had explained that medical charting had begun as a way for doctors to communicate what they found, thought, and did for a patient to the next doctor who happened to see that patient to ensure continuity of care. These days, in the era of electronic medical records, "documentation" seems less about communicating to other clinicians than about covering legalities and getting paid.

I told Alison, a medical student and budding family physician, about Narrative Medicine, a movement championed by Dr. Rita Charon at Columbia University, which seeks to retain the patient's story within the medical encounter. I explained to Alison that while some of what we do, such as adjusting pain medications, can be adequately recorded in template notes, I was determined to resist the dehumanizing influence of "spreadsheet charting." When visits involve decision-making and counseling, I often scribble quotes while I am in the room as a way of capturing the dynamics and conveying the essence of what took place. It is an effort to preserve the personhood of the patient and protect the soul of medicine within the notes I write.

In Sharon's case, I also used narrative charting and pasted in e-mail exchanges between Stephanie and me to convey the sequence of conversations and decision-making, as they unfolded, to Dr. Ruiz and the other specialists involved in Sharon's care. Partly, I felt it was important for them to know that I didn't talk her or her mother into anything, but supported them in making their own decisions—at their own pace, to the extent that was possible.

Outpatient Challenges were now complete and the morning meeting's agenda moved on to each of the hospitalized patients before wrapping up. Then Helen, Christopher, Dr. Macy, and I headed out of the office and down the back halls of the hospital to begin making rounds and visiting patients. Alison went with Betty Priest and Laura Rollano to see patients in the clinic. The rest of the morning was fairly unremarkable.

After lunch, just before one thirty in the afternoon, Christopher and I were talking with the family of an elderly man in the emergency department when my pager vibrated on my hip. The display read 33315, which meant that an outside call was holding. Unless I picked up the call, I might not know who was trying to reach me. During weekdays, most calls go through our office; clinical questions go to our triage nurse. But we maintain a twenty-four-hour, just-in-time phone consultation service for physicians in the region. Our flyers instruct physicians to call the main number and ask for the palliative care physician on call. So the person listening to the wait tone could be a physician from somewhere in the region who was calling with a pressing clinical question.

I answered the page from the nearest nursing station and waited for the tone that indicates I was connected. "Hello, this is Dr. Byock."

"Hi, Dr. Byock, this is Millie, Sharon Valero's hospice nurse. I thought you would want to know that Sharon has taken a major turn." She paused before adding, "She is comfortable, but no longer saying much. About eleven a.m., her breathing became more labored. I did turn her oxygen up to five liters per minute and gave her another dose of morphine. She settled down and said she felt better and was able to take a few sips of tea. Now she is curled up on her bed in the living room with her cat. She is starting to mottle in her legs. The family is all here. I don't think it will be long."

Without knowing it, I'd closed my eyes and balanced on my heels, leaning against the nursing station wall, my back straight, breathing in deep, rhythmic fashion. Nurses, interns, residents, transporters, and housekeeping personnel were going about their business, but I was in a bubble. I was not shocked; indeed I had been expecting such a call, but I still dreaded it.

———

I PICTURED Sharon as I had seen her just four days ago. She was sitting cross-legged on a bed that her family had set up in their living room, a red fleece blanket draped around her and a white kitten curled in her lap. It was Friday evening about six thirty; I was returning from my meeting in Chicago and had stopped by on my way home from the airport.

Their home was in a set of row houses in a neighborhood less than a quarter hour's drive from the Manchester, New Hampshire, airport. It took me a few minutes that evening to find their home amid several dozen units with uniform gray siding and black-and-white vertical-striped awnings, many adorned with flower boxes covered in snow and holiday decorations and children's art in the windows. I finally recognized Stephanie's yellow Ford Taurus and her bumper sticker: EACH DAY IS A GIFT FROM GOD. HAVE YOU THANKED HIM LATELY?

I had called on my cell phone from my car, so Stephanie was standing at the front window, wiping away steam and watching for me as I walked to their door. A dense aroma of stew billowed out of the open door. Stephanie looked into my eyes, hugged me, and said, "Thank you so much for coming. It will mean so much to Sharon." As I followed her to the living room, I took note of the steep carpeted staircase that led to the bedrooms and remembered Sharon describing it like an elderly tenant of a fifth-story walk-up. She planned her days around getting up and down those stairs.

Movie posters and Christian art shared limited wall space with open cabinets filled with music CDs, videotapes, and DVDs that gave the room a cluttered feel. The centerpiece of the living room was a large flat-screen television that hung on one wall, with the room's furniture— a love seat, recliner, and Sharon's bed—arranged in an arc for easy viewing. A Patriots game was in the last two minutes; with time-outs and commercials, I guessed the game had another ten or fifteen minutes to go. Bill turned his head, waved, and started to get up, but I insisted that he stay put and quickly crossed the room to shake his good right hand. Behind his recliner hung a poster with a *trompe l'oeil* antique wooden frame surrounding weathered parchment and bearing a handwritten aphorism: "Sometimes God Calms the Storm . . . Sometimes He Lets the Storm Rage and Calms His Child."

Sharon looked pale and exhausted. It seemed an effort for her to keep her head up. As I took her hand and leaned forward, I could hear the whistle of high-flow oxygen from the soft plastic cannulae in her nose.

"How are you doing, kiddo?" I asked.

"Okay," she smiled. "I like being home."

"Are they taking good care of you?" I asked in a teasing tone. The love in the room was thicker than the smell of the simmering stew.

"Yes"—Sharon rolled her eyes—"they are being good to me."

"How are things working out with Millie, your hospice nurse?"

"Good. She's really nice."

I remarked that Snowball, her new cat, seemed to have settled right in.

"She's not my cat," Sharon corrected me. "Chloe was my cat. This cat is a pest," she insisted, faithfully sticking up for her deceased, homely, hairless feline friend as she lovingly stroked Snowball's neck and belly.

Right after I'd referred her to hospice, Sharon's hospice nurse, Millie, had called me, and we reviewed her medications and discussed in detail what treatments, specific medicines, and doses she would have for expected problems of fever, pain, and shortness of breath. In addition to twice-daily methadone, I increased her dose of oral morphine to 15 milligrams up to every hour as needed for breakthrough pain and to reduce any sense of air hunger. Opioid medications, such as morphine, have been shown to decrease the work of breathing—the effort and metabolic energy required to lower the diaphragm, expand the chest, and draw air into the lungs—so that, in addition to comfort, people actually breathe more easily.

Still, it was likely that the medication was contributing to Sharon's fatigue. I suspected that she was forcing herself to stay up until I arrived.

Fortunately, the football game finally ended. Stephanie immediately headed for the kitchen and returned with a tray filled with bowls of homemade beef stew and a freshly baked loaf of bread. Although my wife, Yvonne, and I had planned to have dinner at home later in the evening, I had no thought of declining.

As we ate our stew, we didn't explicitly talk about Sharon's dying, although there was no hint of denial. Instead, we talked about the people who were coming to visit—her father and his wife; her younger brother, Bob, who had been estranged from the family (except for Sharon) for the past few years and often was out of touch for months; her older brother, Eddie, who was serving in the military in Iraq and coming home with assistance from the International Red Cross.

With dinner finished and Sharon looking more and more tired, I said I should probably be getting on my way.

"I will be checking on you," I said, adding, "Your mom and Millie can reach me at any time."

"I know," she said, smiling weakly. She lifted her left arm, inviting me to hug her—which I did. It was her way of giving me permission to leave.

As I drove home, I spoke with each of my daughters on my cell phone, telling them how much I loved them.

MY REVERIE LASTED just a few seconds. With my eyes open, I was back in the hospital, just four days later, aware of my back against the nursing station wall and the hum of activity around me. I thanked Millie for calling, said that I will expect to hear from her again later, and asked her to tell Stephanie they were all in my thoughts.

It was approaching four o'clock when my pager went off again, and once again it was an outside call. This time I expected it would be Millie updating me again. I knew, though still dreaded what was coming.

"Hello, this is Ira," I said as the call went through.

"Hi, Dr. Byock, it's Millie." The somber tone of her voice telegraphed her message. "Well, she is gone."

"Oh," I sighed, unsurprised. "Was she comfortable?"

"Yes, entirely. She simply went to sleep. I was able to get her to take a dose of Tylenol and her morphine. We used a moist towel to help keep her fever down. Stephanie was holding her when she died."

"And how is Stephanie doing?" I asked.

"As well as can be expected. She never left Sharon's side and showered her with affection as she died. Now she's a bit numb, I think. It is still too new and unreal. But her whole family is here. The place is full, which is good for Stephanie. Her minister is here, too. I don't think they will leave her alone for a while. We are awaiting the funeral home people. At the moment they are having a prayer circle over Sharon's body."

I thanked Millie again for calling—and for the tender care she gave Sharon. I ask her to tell Stephanie that I send my sympathies and love, and that I will call her this evening.

I sighed again, feeling the familiar pang of sadness that clenches within my chest whenever I think of Sharon's tragic life. I thought of the emotional highs and lows of the years in which I had known her. Two moments in time stood out.

SHARON RELIGIOUSLY WATCHED Jeff Corwin's show on Animal Planet every weekday afternoon. Woe to anyone who tried to interrupt her when Jeff Corwin was on the tube.

I suggested she write him a letter. "I will make sure he receives it if you write it," I reassured her. After some editing by her mother, a night nurse, and me, here is what Sharon produced:

Dear Jeff,

I have wanted to meet you for a long time. I love to watch
your shows because they brighten my day, especially
when I'm in the hospital. I'm in the hospital a lot because
I have cystic fibrosis and the related problems of diabetes,
osteoporosis, and cirrhosis of the liver.

I love all animals. I am 17. I want to learn about all of
the planet's animals. I have a special love of the ocean and
want to become a marine biologist. I also love snakes and
want to explore becoming a herpetologist.

There are also many other careers I have an interest in
exploring, including being a veterinarian, but I don't want
to take too much time here to write them all down. I think
it's enough to say that I'm more comfortable with animals
than with people.

I would love to meet you because I have many
questions for you and would love to just talk for a few
minutes in person. Is there any way for me to visit with
you, even briefly, at your place in Massachusetts?

Please say Hi to your fox, Tea-cup, for me.

I hope to hear from you.

Best regards,
Sharon Valero

I DID SOME SLEUTHING by Internet and phone, and was able to contact Corwin's publicist, who agreed to put the letter in his hands. He
responded within a day. Not long after, he hosted her during a show he
put on for a fair in Massachusetts, taking her "backstage" and letting
her hold several animals, including Tea-cup. The next day, Stephanie

was breathless over the phone as she told me about Sharon's visit. She said I would not have recognized her daughter—not only because she had shampooed, blow-dried, and brushed her hair, and freshly filed and polished her nails, but because she was shy, quiet, and polite, and "on her very best behavior!"

When I saw Sharon again—it was just two weeks later that she was again admitted to the hospital—she felt physically lousy, but emotionally she was still glowing from the visit. It was "the best day of my life!" she told me. Between spasms of coughing, she smiled and showed me pictures her mother had taken of her with Corwin. I was already beaming when, for the first time in the many months I had known her, she opened her arms and gave me a big hug.

That hug warmed my old doctor's heart, but I suppressed a shiver as I embraced Sharon's emaciated frame and felt my fingers fall into the deep grooves between her ribs.

For me, the lowest point in Sharon's care were the last days she was in the hospital and the discussions I described in her chart, during which Sharon, Stephanie, and I talked about her going home and made plans for how she would be cared for and how she would die. Although I had known it was coming and had been preparing myself for months, I was aware of my own deep-seated desire to delay or defer the conversation. It was as if talking about her dying would make it real. Even in my role as a palliative care doctor, I kept thinking of anything else we could do to prolong her life—and avoid having the conversation.

There was a moment when Sharon helped me through it. Stephanie left to talk with a nurse—and, I suspect, to give Sharon some privacy of a few moments alone with her doctor. I had one unfinished piece of business that had been bothering me.

"Sharon," I said softly, "I have something I need to say. I want to apologize for failing to fatten you up enough to grow breasts. I never forgot what you told me the day we met and, well, I really tried and I am sorry."

Sharon thought I might be making a feeble attempt at a joke and, at first, gave me a "yeah, right" look and ironic smile. But she saw I was sincere and immediately softened.

"It's nobody's fault," she said, letting me off the hook and, more important, forgiving herself.

BEFORE DINNER—it was nearly eight p.m.—I called Stephanie. She answered on the first ring.

"I am so sorry that your precious daughter has died."

"Oh, Ira, I will miss her terribly." She pauses to clear her throat. "I know she is with Jesus," she says. "She was beautiful to the very end. She just snuggled up and went to sleep. We all kissed her and stroked her hair. The last hour or so, she just slowed down and her breaths were further apart. Then she wasn't there. I felt her soul leave her body."

"I will never forget her," I said. "But I sure am glad I got to know her."

"We could not have done this without you, Ira. Sharon loved you, ya know."

"Well, the feeling was mutual."

I asked if there were any funeral plans. Stephanie said that there would be a memorial "celebration of life" the coming Sunday at two p.m. at their church in Goffstown.

"I hope you can be there," she said. I told her that I would be.

Part Five

Transforming Medicine and Society

8.

Fixing Health Care

Ira, the nurse at Mom's Alzheimer's unit just called. They sent her to the hospital yesterday afternoon—said that she'd been vomiting and there was nothing else they could do. They didn't even call me! Damn it! She even hates to be touched and now she is strapped to a gurney in some emergency room, getting X-rays and IVs."

Despite a lousy cell phone connection, I could hear tears within the tremble of my friend Michelle's voice. I knew something was wrong from the number on my cell phone's display, even before I flipped it open. Michelle would never call my cell on a weekday morning unless something bad had happened. Now, she hadn't paused to say hello, and I understood from her pace and anxious tone that she'd been talking to me before I'd answered the phone.

"I'm just sick about it. I'm not mad at you, Ira, but I did everything you suggested and none of it worked. Naturally, her own doctor's not on call. I'm still trying to find the doctor who is.

What should I do now?!"

Michelle is married to a close boyhood friend of mine, and my wife and I have been good friends of theirs for many years. Michelle owns and directs an executive search firm based in Manhattan. She is meticulous and exacting in her business and personal life, as confident and assertive as anyone I know. Michelle is also an accomplished artist with a keen aesthetic sense that extends to cooking, home decor, and adventurous travel. She is an attractive brunette who is nearly a decade younger than her husband and I. Her disciplined commitment to eating right and a regular, strenuous exercise program keep her fit and able to enjoy long hours.

Over the eleven years from the earliest onset of her mother's cognitive decline, to the day of Michelle's call, she and I often talked about her mother's condition and she sought my advice in planning her mother's health care. Michelle felt a keen responsibility for her mother's well-being and was determined for her to receive the best possible care. We usually spoke informally over dinners with our spouses—parent care is a common topic of dinner conversations among couples our age—but sometimes she brought a list of questions and had a pen in hand as we more formally considered details of her mother's functional abilities, emotional well-being, living situation, and medical plans. As her mother's dementia accelerated and she became progressively debilitated, Michelle and I occasionally spoke by phone in the evening, discussing changes in her mother's condition or the pros and cons of various medications or treatments.

Her mother, Jeanne Gider, was a remarkable individual. She was a retired physician who had come to medicine as a second career. Born in Brooklyn in 1929, Jeanne Goldberg grew up during the Depression and the lean years of World War II. At age thirteen she wrote in her diary that she wanted to become a doctor. However, limited family finances and her gender led to nursing school instead. She became a public health nurse, a nursing instructor, and then earned a master's in public administration from New York University. She married Leo Stuhl, an agricultural economist who had worked on the Aswan Dam, but was subsequently blacklisted from government jobs during the McCarthy era. The couple moved to Toledo, Ohio. Leo became a traveling sales-man of toys and confections, and Jeanne became the director of nursing at Flower Hospital. In 1955 Leo became ill with cancer. Surprisingly, while he underwent cancer treatments that might have rendered him infertile, Michelle was conceived. Leo Stuhl lived to see his daughter born and grow to age two. But Michelle's father never regained his health and died in 1959.

Suddenly a young widow, Jeanne and little Michelle moved to Miami to be closer to Leo's aging mother. Jeanne took a job as a technician in a local medical laboratory. It wasn't long before the supervising physi-cian of the laboratory recognized Jeanne's intellect and ambition, and began encouraging her to go to medical school. Her family was able and eager to help. Applying to medical school in 1965 as a woman who was nearly a decade older than most applicants seemed a herculean feat. Against long odds, she was accepted—one of only four women in her University of Miami Medical School class—and at age thirty-two she followed her long-held dream.

After completing her training in 1971, Jeanne remarried and went on to become a busy family practitioner and respected member of the south Florida medical community. As a family doctor, Jeanne Gider was skilled in helping people plan for the end of life. She even served for several years as a volunteer member of the board of directors of a local hospice program. Michelle said that her mother had long been vocal with her about what she personally wanted—and, mostly, didn't want—as she was dying.

During years of practice, Dr. Gider had seen many difficult deaths that she thought were the consequences of doctors and family members trying to prolong life at all costs. She made Michelle promise not to allow that to happen to her. After her second marriage ended in divorce, she prepared an advance directive document that named Michelle, her only child, as her authorized medical decision-maker. In the document, Jeanne specified that if she had a life-threatening illness and was too

ill to speak for herself, she did not want any invasive measures to prolong her life: no surgery, no CPR, no mechanical ventilation, no artificial
nutrition and hydration.

In 1984, Jeanne was in a serious car accident in which she suffered
a concussion. After months of outpatient rehabilitation she was able to
function well enough to work as a medical consultant and lecturer to
hospitals for several years. However, she never returned to providing
direct clinical care. Then, in 1991, at age sixty-two, she was diagnosed
with colon cancer and underwent surgery. Although she was apparently
cured of her cancer, her recovery coincided with an accelerated progression of dementia. For the next few years, while the disease was still
in the early and middle stages, Jeanne was able to feed and dress herself.
During this period, in one of our conversations, I suggested to Michelle
that she make an appointment with her mother's doctor specifically to
develop contingency plans for foreseeable future problems. She thought
it was a great idea.

At the appointment a few weeks later, Michelle and her mother's
internist sat in his office and reviewed Jeanne's advance directive.
Michelle discussed the conversations she had had with her mother. The
doctor readily agreed that the sole focus of her mother's care would
be her comfort and quality of life. He understood that if and when a
complication of her illness occurred, it was Michelle's intention to allow
her to die naturally. Michelle was explicit that her mother was not to be
hospitalized without her permission. Again, the doctor fully agreed. He
placed Michelle's contact information—including her cell phone, pager,
and home numbers—prominently in her mother's chart. Michelle told
me that she saw the numbers on a face sheet within the manila card-
board folder that held her mother's clinical records.

The next time we spoke, Michelle thanked me for making the suggestion. She felt confident having her mother's doctor on board with her
mother's wishes.

Because her mother wanted to stay in her own home in south Florida for as long as possible—and because they had the financial means to do so—for nearly eight years Michelle hired aides and coordinated her mother's home care. During those years, she says, "Mom was able to participate in the world" and enjoy most days. The pace of her decline quickened, and by 1999 Jeanne required around-the-clock supervision. In addition, at times she became agitated with apparent paranoid delusions. Michelle carefully evaluated every specialized dementia care facility in the region and, after frantic weeks of waiting lists, her mother was admitted to the one she felt was best. (Michelle once quipped that it was as hard for her mother to get into a good nursing home as it had been to get into medical school.)

Admission to the specialized nursing home came just in time but proved to have been worth the wait. Within months, Jeanne was barely communicating, completely disoriented, and in diapers. She spent most of her days sitting in a chair in the day room. She no longer recognized Michelle or anyone else. She was mostly placid, but recoiled from being touched. Unless the nurse aides who knew her well were oh-so-gentle and soothing in their approach, she would recoil and become agitated when they tried to bathe her or provide daily mouth care.

ON THE DAY of her frantic call, despite all of Michelle's meticulous efforts—and my supposedly expert guidance—her mother was a captive, tied down and undergoing a battery of unwanted blood tests, X-rays, and treatments. Indeed "battery" seemed the right word.

What should she do now?

My advice was simple, though not easy. I told her to fly down to Miami immediately. "Until you're convinced she's safe, do not leave your mother alone." I was speaking literally and she knew it.

Late that evening, Michelle called from her mother's hospital bedside. She had caught an afternoon flight from New York and touched down about eight p.m. Her mother was much as she had feared—bruised from the IVs and blood tests, with cotton restraints tied around each of her ankles and anchored to a bedpost. She was sedated but, when aroused, obviously confused and visibly uncomfortable.

"Get this," Michelle plaintively exclaimed over the phone, "I reached the doctor on call as I was packing to leave for the airport. He said they had to hospitalize her because she has an obstructed bowel and might have cancer. So I asked him, 'What the hell are you going to do if she has cancer?' and he said, 'Well, she'd need surgery.' I told him in no uncertain terms that under *no circumstances* would I consent to any surgery for my mother. I demanded that my mom be made comfortable and hinted strongly that I was willing to sue him and the nursing home if he didn't follow my instructions. He sounded surprised, but also relieved, 'Oh, okay, we'll focus on her comfort, and I guess we should arrange for hospice,' he said."

He got that right. In fact, there are ways of controlling the discomfort bowel obstructions cause without surgery, but doing so would take palliative care expertise of the sort that a hospice program provides.

At Michelle's direction, and with the on-call doctor's blessing, her mother was transferred from the hospital to a hospice inpatient facility across the street. For the last ten days of her life, there were no restraints on her arms or legs. She was in no distress, thanks to sufficient medication for pain and anxiety. Her mouth was moist and her skin was clean, warm, and dry. The hospice staff treated Jeanne Gider tenderly, respected her dignity, and enabled her to die peacefully.

The story would have been sobering and instructive had it ended there, but it didn't.

A month after Jeanne died, Michelle received a bill for her mother's twenty-three-hour hospitalization. It totaled $22,402. (Adjusted for inflation, the amount would exceed $27,000 in 2012.) The bill included $6,750 for twenty-two separate blood tests, $1,077 for three electrocardiograms, $4,187 for a CAT scan of her head, $776 for three X-rays of her abdomen, $296 for a chest X-ray, and $3,246 for three ultrasound tests.

Michelle was stunned and called the billing department to complain. Anger, which had been smoldering within her grief, threatened to erupt. The clerk went over the itemized statement and assured her that the charges were correct. Michelle first told the billing clerk and then a supervisor that the bill was outrageous, explaining that the tests and treatments her mother received were unauthorized and unwanted. Michelle was spoiling for an argument, but there was none to be had. The customer service specialist calmly let Michelle know that she needn't worry. "This will not be a problem," she said. "Medicare will pay."

NOT A PROBLEM?

What happened to my friend and her mother is not just one story. Their experiences are emblematic of the health care system we have. What makes Jeanne Gider's dying stand out for me is the lengths to which Michelle had gone to prevent these needless, intrusive medical treatments and how, in the end, it hadn't worked. The story of what happened to her mother is a cautionary tale for all of us who have aging parents or who happen to be aging ourselves.

Notice that in this saga there was no malevolence on anyone's part. Despite good intentions and the careful planning Michelle had done, when her mother developed abdominal pain and vomiting, thereby categorically shifting from being "chronically ill" to "acutely ill," the acute care system snapped into action. As if a valve had opened, a cascade of events was released. No one stopped to check her advance directive or call Michelle, her legal decision-maker. Instead, clinical protocols and patterned responses of nurses, doctors, health care facilities, and teams were set in motion, forming a swift current that carried Jeanne Gider to the hospital. Doctors and nurses with long-standing habits generated routine tests and instituted acute treatments. With practiced handoffs, Jeanne was passed from the nursing home staff to EMTs to emergency department staff, to the on-call physician internist and surgeon, and to the hospital nurses. Once unleashed, the current was difficult to stop. No wonder Michelle felt she was swimming upstream.

This tragic tale illustrates the systemic challenges we face and highlights the urgent need to revise care standards and redesign health care systems. We must do so in order to protect vulnerable patients—our parents, grandparents, spouses, brothers, and sisters. And we must do so to ensure that our children are not left in Michelle's predicament, struggling to protect their parents and feeling guilty for being unable to keep their promises to us.

Not every frail elder or dying person has as strong and sophisticated an advocate as Michelle. As they approach the end of life, people are at risk of suffering needlessly from lapses in communication, failures of coordination, and missing preparations for foreseeable crises. When things fall apart, often patients and their families don't know what to do. Calling 911, while understandable, is not always the best answer.

As broken as our national and local health care systems are now, we may soon be nostalgic for these times. We are on the cusp of a national crisis that will affect every person in America. Like a tsunami in slow motion, demographic tides of frailty and physical illness are rising, not just "nationally" in some abstract sense, but in each of our own communities. You likely know people who are sick or frail who live just across the street or down the block or in your apartment building. Even today, there's a good chance those people and their families are hard put to deal with their daily medical care. Many are also struggling to meet their basic needs. As hard as things are today, the crisis is merely beginning. It is time we developed plans to deal with it.

And we can. Today, we have the knowledge and expertise available to respond in effective ways. Many thousands of experiences like Jeanne Gider's have provided data for researchers in public health, geriatrics, sociology, and palliative care to analyze and make sense of. We know where the cracks lie in our health and social architecture of caring.

More important, creative researchers, advocates, and innovators within these fields have developed strategies for fixing the fractures.

A common assumption among politicians and social commentators is that budget woes are keeping us from providing the best possible care for people at the end of life. In reality, few people in medicine, sociology, or health services research who have studied the situation agree with that premise. In fact, our society has had the technical knowledge and professional expertise we need for some time. But knowing and doing are two different things. What is most worrisome today is that caring well for people through the end of life and supporting caregivers are still not on the national agenda. The clock is ticking along with 78 million baby boomers' beating hearts, but the body politic isn't listening.

In 1997 the Institute of Medicine published *Approaching Death*, a landmark report that surveyed all the available evidence pertinent to dying in America. *Approaching Death* cited widespread "errors of omission and commission" in end-of-life care. Studies found that pain was inconsistently assessed and often poorly treated. Communication around end-of-life planning and preferences often did not occur. Treatments were often given when there was little chance of success but every chance of increasing a patient's distress. Reimbursement systems incentivized treating disease ("at all costs"), as did a legal system that placed physicians at more risk for doing too little than for doing too much. The Institute of Medicine described pervasive deficiencies in medical and nursing education. In its report the institute issued a call for dramatic improvements in clinicians' training, as well as in health services and systems of care, and in community-based responses for people approaching the end of life.

Since *Approaching Death* was published, numerous professional associations and patient advocacy groups have joined the call to vastly improve—indeed to redesign—our nation's medical and social systems to provide the safe, reliable, coordinated, individualized services to ill and elderly people and their families.

So far, it hasn't happened. The dominant social response to illness and frailty remains purely medical. Once one has a diagnosis or two—*bona fide* physical and mental ailments—society will pay for treatments. That's well and good. However, the diagnosis-driven, narrowly defined social response to people's needs misses opportunities for preventing illness, alleviating distress, and enhancing people's well-being. And the exclusively disease- and treatment-oriented nature of contemporary medicine causes dissatisfaction for patients and providers alike.

It is one of the reasons that doctors are burning out in unprecedented numbers. Physician satisfaction with their careers is at an all-time low. Rates of depression, drug abuse, and divorce are higher among physicians than the general public. Today's doctors practice under the scrutiny of business managers, payers, quality committees, and regulators. They feel pressured to see too many patients in too little time. Although physicians tend to be cautious and conscientious by nature, in the United States malpractice suits are always in the back of their minds. In settings in which care is episodic and continuity difficult to assure, all of these factors—feeling pressured and being cautious, conscientious, and concerned about being sued—contribute to doctors' decisions to order extra blood tests, CT scans, and MRI scans, "to be on the safe side."

Patients, especially older patients, also feel rushed and are often left with the impression that their doctors have precious little time or attention for them. It is increasingly common for medical records to be electronic, and in many of the most modern medical centers, doctors spend more time looking at computer screens than at the people sitting in front of them.

People with chronic, life-threatening conditions commonly find that their care feels fragmented and that their doctors aren't communicating with one another. When a patient sees a medical consultant or surgeon, at times key test results or scans aren't available; sometimes tests must be repeated because results of even recent blood work or scans can't be found. When patients ask about the chances of a new treatment working or how long they may have to live, their doctors may be evasive. Doctors who listen carefully, and who consistently answer questions fully, stand out as glowing exceptions in the opinions of many seniors. But they are uncommon in systems fixated on diagnosing and treating pathologies rather than people.

In the current systems and professional culture of medicine, planning, preventing, guidance, and counseling are ancillary and easily ignored. Insurers, Medicare, and Medicaid more readily pay for diagnosing and treating diseases than anything else that doctors do. If complications of treatments occur, these new problems (aka diagnoses) generate more tests and treatments, which are also paid for. Of late, Medicare has refused to pay hospitals the full costs of care for patients who are readmitted within a month of discharge for the same condition. But in general, the government and insurance companies have simply paid.

Like everyone else in the workforce these days, physicians are accountable for what they do. Rightly so. Unfortunately, what they are held accountable for has usually emphasized volume over quality. Physician economic productivity is measured in work RVUs, which stands for relative value units. RVUs accrue through both the time and the intensity or sophistication of specific services. Invasive procedures, such as operations, endoscopies, repairing lacerations, and reducing fractures, are assigned many more RVUs of service than visits to counsel patients and families through difficult, complex decisions or to help them cope with progressive, incurable conditions. Each physician's RVUs are measured and a doctor's output—per day, per month, and per year—can be compared to national benchmarks or local peers and used in performance reviews, yearly bonuses, and salary adjustments. Whether or not their own incomes are affected by how many RVUs they generate, doctors are aware that the more time they spend with patients in talking and counseling, the less revenue their practice generates.

While revenue can rise or fall, overhead tends to be fixed. Physicians in group practices particularly feel the weight of their practices' "overhead," which represents the livelihoods of the managers, nurses, lab techs, receptionists, secretaries, and billing clerks with whom they work. All things being equal, practices succeed when physicians see more patients per unit of time. Yes, doctors can get paid for home visits. And seeing patients in their homes is desirable in some ways—assessments may be more meaningful and treatment plans better fitted to the patient and family's living situation. But in the world of RVUs, unless a patient happens to live across the hall from the physician's office, it is not an efficient use of a doctor's time. Similarly, care planning meetings, and calls and e-mails among providers (social workers and home health or hospice nurses)—the very stuff of coordinated care—detract from physician productivity. For many doctors, it is not a question of income as much as social responsibility to their employees and coworkers within the existing payment system that motivates them to see as many patients as they feasibly can.

A typical internist or family practitioner is scheduled to see ten or more patients in each half day of his or her clinic or office practice. New patient visits are typically scheduled for thirty to forty-five minutes and follow-up patients as little as fifteen. As long as the patients are all generally healthy and the visits are for a yearly health evaluation, or for treatment for high blood pressure, or for weight loss, or to start or adjust medication for depression—and if the doctor is experienced and highly efficient—this level of productivity is achievable. But for many of us—myself included—it is a dizzying pace. When even a few of a doctor's patients have multiple medical problems and chronic conditions—diabetes, hypertension, obesity, congestive heart failure, AND depression—and are taking eight different medications, those fifteen-minute visits are just not enough time. Not even close.

Of course, on any given day, when a physician may be scheduled to see twenty or more patients in the office or clinic, it is also likely one or more of the practice's patients will develop an acute problem and need to be seen. One patient may be an older man with metastatic cancer who has become sedentary over the past two months and now has a cough and fever. Another patient may be a woman with moderate dementia who lives in a nursing home and now has abdominal pain and vomiting and is agitated.

Trying to manage the myriad problems of a chronically ill patient in a busy office practice can feel like juggling Jell-O on a busy city street corner in a rainstorm.

The easiest, safest, and most efficient thing for a doctor to do is to send such acutely ill patients to the hospital. Once there, emergency department or hospital internal medicine physicians and nurses can take over and skillfully order the right tests and treatments for the patients' medical problems.

Doctors know that if they send a patient "to the E.D.," they will be called by the emergency physician, updated, and likely asked for advice. If the patient needs to be admitted, in most hospitals, a hospital internal medicine physician will manage the acute problem. The doctor can visit the patient in the hospital after office hours or the next morning.

In an ideal world, the doctor would be able to urgently see patients who are chronically ill and have now become acutely ill, with their families, before admitting them to a hospital. The doctor, patient, and family would discuss what the turn of events means in light of a person and family's goals of care. What should the balance be now between treatments to save and prolong life and the person's comfort? Is going into the hospital acceptable or should we try to treat this new problem at home or in the nursing home? Would they put any limits on life-prolonging treatments if he suddenly became much worse? How important is it to preserve the opportunity to die naturally?

In the real world, doing what feels clinically right in such situations could easily consume an hour of time. In a busy clinic or medical office this would result in keeping other, scheduled patients waiting—annoying at least a few—and leave a responsible doctor feeling irresponsible to other patients, as well as to his or her practice partners and staff.

Money does not drive the health care system. Money fuels it. When someone is seriously injured or ill, everybody in the system strives to get the person well. Money is no object—it is purely instrumental to getting all the treatments people need.

In the presence of so many problems and needs, everyone at ground level—patients, their families, and physicians—reflexively assumes that the more medical care they can give or receive, the better. There is now compelling evidence disproving that assumption.

Over two decades of research by Drs. John Wennberg, Elliott Fisher, and colleagues at The Dartmouth Institute for Health Policy and Clinical Practice documents large variations in the types and amounts of health care people receive during the last year of life. Analyzing Medicare data, the researchers found substantial differences from one part of the country to another in the number of days spent in hospitals and ICUs, specialists seen, and invasive procedures performed during the last year of life. Drilling into the data, they found striking differences in patterns of care between one city and another even within the same state, and sometimes between one major medical center and another in the same city.

Each edition of the *Dartmouth Atlas of Health Care* has found that greater intensities of medical services correspond with higher costs, but not with longer survival or better health outcomes. Despite seeing more specialists, undergoing more tests, and having more treatments, people who have cancer, heart attacks, or fractured hips—and reside where high medical intensity is the norm—don't live measurably better or longer than people in regions of lower medical intensity. In fact, in areas accustomed to more medical and surgical treatments for these conditions, patients have comparatively poorer functional outcomes and lower satisfaction with care. When it comes to the final years of their lives, people in higher-intensity regions and institutions spend more of their time in hospitals and ICUs and less of their time at home.

When they looked at the academic medical centers that were ranked highest by *U.S. News and World Report*, the *Dartmouth Atlas* researchers found that average costs during the last two years of life ranged from $93,842 per patient at UCLA Medical Center in Los Angeles to $53,432 at Mayo Clinic in Minnesota. Mayo Clinic doctors were hardly skimping on treatments, yet were able to provide what they felt was the best care for patients at nearly half the cost of their colleagues at UCLA.

This is more than an economic issue. Quality of care also varies among institutions and regions, and access to needed health services can be limited. One example that is relevant for people with cancer is access to hospice services, which for many represents the best care for the end of life. This is not merely my assertion as a proud clinician in the field. The Institute of Medicine and the American Society of Clinical Oncology, among many other professional bodies, have called for expanding hospice use among people with late-stage cancer. Still, cancer patients in the United States today have little better than a fifty-fifty chance of receiving hospice care during the last month of their lives. Within that national average, the likelihood of being referred for hospice care varies widely from place to place. For instance, in a November 2010 *Dartmouth Atlas Project* report, "Quality of End-of-life Cancer Care for Medicare Beneficiaries," people with incurable cancers treated at New York's Montefiore Medical Center in the Bronx or Westchester Medical Center in Valhalla have just an 18.6 percent chance of receiving hospice care, while someone with the same condition treated at Monmouth Medical Center in Long Branch, New Jersey, had a 73 percent chance—a nearly fourfold difference in cities that are a car ride apart.

The under-referral and underutilization of hospice care is a serious problem for people dying of cancer. Even in the highest-referring regions and medical centers, they are referred to hospice very late in the course of their illnesses and lives. When Congress passed the Medicare Hospice Benefit in 1982, the law anticipated that people would, on average, receive six months of hospice care before they died. Lawmakers understood that some people would receive hospice care for just a few days and that some would appropriately receive hospice care for substantially longer than six months. They designed the hospice benefit with provisions for mandatory reevaluation and recertification every three months after the initial six months of hospice service. Instead, year after year, the national median length of hospice service ranges from sixteen to twenty days, and many dying people receive hospice care for fewer than three days. Intended as high-quality end-of-life care, for many patients hospice has become brink-of-death care. Not surprisingly, in geographic regions and cancer centers in which patients receive fewer days of hospice care, they spend relatively more time in hospitals and undergo more tests and treatments in the days before death.

Michelle's mother lived in the most medically expensive area in the country, a dubious distinction that has not changed appreciably in the years since Jeanne Gider died. According to the *Dartmouth Atlas of Health Care*, in Miami, someone with a chronic illness has a 30 percent chance of spending time in an ICU at the end of life. This is more than twice the likelihood of dying in an ICU that someone who is living with the same condition in Portland, Oregon, would have.

The historical old saw, "Geography is destiny," turns out to hold true in modern America.

Harvard surgeon and *New Yorker* magazine staff writer Atul Gawande set out to get a sense of why the regional disparities described in the *Dartmouth Atlas* occurred. He visited McAllen, Texas, which ranks among the highest in per capita health care expenses in the country. Care during the last year of life in McAllen, Texas, costs Medicare on average double what it does about eight hundred miles north in El Paso, and two and a quarter times what it does in Rochester, Minnesota.

Treatment in McAllen is not bad; by several parameters, it is quite good. The town is replete with medical and surgical specialists and can deliver state-of-the-art treatments for cancer and heart disease. People receive a lot of care, more than in most American cities. The local medical culture holds that when there is something you can do that might help a patient's condition, and will likely do no harm, why not give it a try? McAllen's doctors are not overtly driven by a profit motive, but since Medicare and insurance companies pay for diagnostic tests and disease treatments, there is no disincentive to doing more.

Many of the doctors and local health system administrators that Dr. Gawande talked with were surprised that their town's practices were so different than El Paso's. They wondered if their patients were more ill or the care they provided was just better. The data show that neither is true. Much more likely, a combination of the McAllen community's ready acceptance of high-intensity treatments and the examples of local physician peers, doing more has come to represent good medical practice there. And like everywhere else, physicians who move to McAllen soon adopt local patterns of practice.

A factor more insidious than efficiency or profit leads doctors to emphasize high-intensity treatments over poignant conversations and counseling, shared decision-making, care planning, and end-of-life care: their aversion to talking about dying and death. Any doctor who dreads talking to patients about dying—and that describes a large majority— quickly learns that ordering more tests and treatments allows him or her to refocus on the disease and sidestep in-depth discussions with patients and their families about these morbid (or mortal) subjects.

Individually, doctors can be excused for these problematic practices. The education system has failed them and the health systems they work in are (with few exceptions) dysfunctional. Collectively, however, the medical profession has some explaining to do to the American public. It is high time that American doctors take a hard look at the reasons we do what we do.

In addition to pointing out problems, the *Dartmouth Atlas* group's body of research identifies bright rays of hope.

Best-performing institutions and regions offer examples to emulate, in the form of practical strategies and model programs we can adopt or adapt to our local systems. High-functioning, lower-cost health care systems are not rare; we know exactly where they are and can learn from them. They can be found in Seattle, Washington; Salt Lake City, Utah; Grand Junction, Colorado; Danville, Pennsylvania; Temple, Texas; Durham, North Carolina; Mason City, Iowa; and Rochester, Minnesota. These systems and leading institutions do not skimp on services or accept lower quality. Instead, they exemplify individualized, patient-centered care. Their secret is no secret at all. Each patient's medical records are kept secure, but also made reliably, readily accessible by doctors involved in the person's care. Emphasis is placed on clear communication, proactive planning, and coordinating care among doctors and other health care providers and teams. More conversation and closer follow-up allows for less *just-to-be-sure* testing. It turns out that another way *to be sure* is *to be in touch*. More collaborative planning and team-to-team communication make for smoother transitions of care from home to hospital to rehabilitation and nursing facilities and back to home with home health or hospice. Communication and planning also result in fewer crises.

The *Dartmouth Atlas* group estimated that Medicare could reduce hospital costs by 28 to 43 percent by adopting the patient-centered, proactive approaches of the most efficient health systems. When he was director of the Office of Management and Budget, Peter Orzag estimated that Medicare could save nearly 30 percent of costs if our nation's health systems operated like the lowest-cost systems.

Care at the end of life will remain expensive, first, because of the continual advances in lifesaving technologies and, second, because people are sickest before they die. Yet with ongoing communication and iterative, proactive decision-making and planning as a person's condition and treatment priorities change, care will less often be astronomically expensive. One multicenter study of eight acute-care hospitals with mature Palliative Care Services compared patients served by palliative care to matched controls. Among patients who received palliative care, costs were $279 less per day and $1,696 less per admission for those who were discharged from the hospital and $374 less per day and $4,908 less per admission for those who died. A similar study of patients in New York State whose hospital bills were paid by Medicaid found that, among patients receiving palliative care, costs were $4,098 less per admission for those discharged alive and $7,563 less for patients who died during the admission than for comparable controls.

These savings occurred in absence of any requirement to forgo treatments or any financial cap on the amount of treatments a patient could receive. In fact, the cost savings were not even intentional. Instead, the lower costs were merely a by-product of palliative care: the result of assiduously matching people's values and preferences to achievable health goals and making those goals the focus of individualized plans of care.

I have known many patients with advanced, incurable conditions who, prior to meeting me or our palliative care team, had assumed that the only choice they had was either accepting every treatment possible or accepting the worst thing possible: death. Before our team became involved, they were never asked whether, in addition to wanting to live as long and as well as possible, they eventually wanted to die gently. Until we met them, they had never been asked where they wanted to be during their last days of life. So, as they became sicker they went to the hospital—and continued to say yes to whatever life-extending treatments were offered.

Although continued innovation is welcome, we no longer have to invent ways to achieve reliable, safe, effective, and efficient care for people through the end of life. Workable and highly affordable strategies for making dramatic, necessary improvements to our nation's health care system exist. We merely have to bring them to scale. But transforming America's broken health care systems will take political will and cultural leadership. For the magnitude of change that is needed to occur, social activism is necessary.

Activism related to elder care and end-of-life care evokes images of silver-haired citizens wearing AARP or Gray Panther T-shirts, demonstrating on the steps of a courthouse, state house, or the Capitol, holding pickets and shouting slogans. And to an extent, political demonstrations and public events of that sort are needed.

Indeed, it is a wonder that the sorry state of dying in America has not sparked a citizen-consumer uproar. Remember Howard Beale, the evening news anchor in the movie *Network*, who exhorted viewers to open their windows and scream, "I'm mad as hell and I'm not going to take it anymore!"? Throughout the city, people threw open their windows and declared their defiance.

In the real world, too, people have often pushed back when they were not getting the care they deserved and organized politically active social movements.

In the 1970s hemodialysis for kidney failure was limited and "God Squad" committees in hospitals decided which patients would receive this life-prolonging treatment. Outcries from people with kidney disease and their families stirred Congress to adopt a special Medicare benefit for dialysis care. When people were dying of AIDS by the thousands, it was citizen activism and voter pressure that drove funding for HIV research. The Ryan White Comprehensive AIDS Resources Emergency (CARE) Act saved millions from dying of HIV-AIDS in the United States. When HMOs and insurance companies were forcing mothers and their newborn infants to leave hospitals within twenty-four hours after giving birth, a combination of consumer and citizen activism swiftly pushed passage of laws and changes in regulations that made "drive-by deliveries" history.

Why not in this situation? Dying is the most universal and arguably most difficult of life events. Pretty much by definition, dying people are as sick as they have ever been. They feel vulnerable—they *are* vulnerable—and many worry about being a burden. Their families are dealing with the strain of caregiving and the pain of losing a loved one who is not yet gone. Given the widespread nature of the deficiencies in care and social support—exemplified by people in pain, rampant rates of medical bankruptcy, nursing homes with too few nurses and aides to take basic care of people—and the toll these rents in the social fabric takes on sick people and their families, one wonders where the public outcry has been. What would it take to evoke a Howard Beale moment?

Of course, dying is different from birthing. It is different from "merely" needing dialysis, or even living with AIDS. For one thing, there is no community of dying people. Dying people die, and caregivers disperse, leaving no base for social or political action. Being mortal is too broad a category to generate a special interest group. There is no membership organization for dying people. (Can you imagine the ads for such a group?)

In addition to feeling too weak, tired, and generally unwell to advocate loudly for themselves, in my experience it is common for dying people to feel vaguely embarrassed about their condition. It is another effect of our death-defying culture. Doctors refer to dying patients as having "failed" medical treatment. (It always seemed to me that it was the treatments that failed the patients!) People come to believe they brought their disease upon themselves by smoking or drinking, or having sex with the wrong people, living in the wrong place, or simply by being too stressed. Similarly, family caregivers—in addition to being too emotionally and physically exhausted to advocate on behalf of their dying relatives and friends—may also feel vaguely insecure and wonder if they are doing all they can or should for the person who is ill. And families do not want to anger the doctors and nurses, or make waves with hospitals and insurance companies they rely on.

Of course, the majority of Americans who are not seriously ill—or currently caring for a frail family member—don't want to think about it. Eventually, when things get bad enough and people get angry enough, we will get over our resistance and get on with fixing the problems. Improving the way we die is, after all, in everyone's self-interest.

History strongly suggests that a combination of citizen and consumer activism will be required to achieve large-scale changes in care systems and patterns of behavior. The collective citizen and consumer efforts to reduce deaths from motor vehicle accidents offer some precedence. Citizens and consumers came together to demand safer cars (air bags and crash safety standards) and safer drivers (Mothers Against Drunk Drivers, stiff DUI [driving under the influence] penalties, Friends Don't Let Friends Drive Drunk, Designated Driver programs). The sciences—epidemiology, surgery, preventive medicine, and public health—called attention to the problem and contributed to solutions. But it was the social movement, people working in concert and taking action in political arenas and the marketplace, that drove dramatic changes.

Voting with one's dollars is a common and (usually) uncontentious form of activism. Customers directly reward businesses, including hospitals, group practices, clinics, home health agencies, and hospices, that provide high-quality services. In recent years CMS (the Centers for Medicare and Medicaid Services), the federal agency that runs Medicare, has published (on the medicare.gov website) report cards with quality ratings of hospitals, nursing homes, and home health agencies. The U.S. Department of Veterans Affairs' Veterans Administration transparently publishes health outcomes achieved by VA medical centers (at HospitalCompare.va.gov) with regard to blood pressure control, diabetes care, heart disease, serious infections, and deaths. Quality data is the fundamental ingredient of consumer activism and a powerful lever for bringing about change. (Data geeks are the unsung heroes of modern social change.)

The more people know about how hospitals, nursing homes, and home health and hospice services perform, the better able we are to vote at the ballot box and in the marketplace. Information about patient-centered aspects of care, such as how well clinical staff listen and communicate and how effectively they manage pain, can drive people to choose one facility or agency over another. Already several websites, like HealthGrades.com, post quality measures about doctors by region and specialty. HealthGrades.com compiles ratings that include how well the doctor listens, how much time he or she spends with patients, and the level of trust the doctor engenders. Doctors can also be compared by surgical outcomes and rates of infections or other complications, as well as by their patients' satisfaction with pain treatment and communication. Such information will be increasingly available. Having health care systems and doctors compete for business on the basis of quality can accelerate needed changes.

Professionals and consumer coalitions can support effective social movements and citizen-consumer advocacy by teaching people what they can expect and how to get it.

The Patient's Bill of Rights and the American Hospital Association's brochure "The Patient Care Partnership" list basic expectations people can have of hospitals and health systems. We have a right to expect that hospitals will be clean and safe places and that the care hospitals give will be high quality. We have a right to a choice of competent providers. We must be given access to emergency services and be treated fairly and with respect. We must have opportunities to take part in medical decisions and can expect that our personal information will be kept private. We are within our rights to expect help when we are discharged from the hospital. And, when needed, we deserve assistance with making sense of medical bills and with arranging reasonable payment plans.

Correspondingly, as patients, we have basic responsibilities. It is our responsibility to be honest and forthcoming with our physicians and other providers. We must participate in decisions about our care—or designate someone we trust to participate for us—and adhere to treatment plans. We are responsible for letting our doctors know when our condition worsens or if we are unable to follow through on treatments. That includes letting our physicians know if we are, or become, unable to pay for medications they prescribe. Finally, we are responsible for making good-faith efforts to pay health care bills and working with providers when we cannot pay in full.

I have my own list of reasonable expectations that patients who are seriously ill deserve to have fulfilled.

To have one's pain and other physical symptoms regularly assessed and competently treated.

To have adequate information about one's condition and treatments, in clear and simple terms.

To have care coordinated between visits and among physicians and health programs involved in one's care.

To have crises prevented when possible and have clear plans for managing emergencies in place.

To have enough nurses and aides on staff in hospitals and nursing homes to provide safe and high-quality care.

To have one's family supported in giving care, in their own strain, and, eventually, in their grief.

Choosing a well-regarded physician and highly rated hospital or health care agency is important, but not sufficient. People have to take responsibility for speaking up for themselves and the people they love. The Patient's Bill of Rights and my list of reasonable expectations are intended to help.

I often suggest to people that they can consider their relationship with their physician as a partnership. Within this partnership they can responsibly advocate for themselves or their loved one. I advise people to keep a running list of questions for their doctors and to keep logs or journals of times that symptoms occur, what they were doing just before the symptoms occurred, as well as what, if anything, they did to alleviate the symptoms, including any medicines they took and how effective the medicines were.

In managing pain, I teach patients a 0-to-10 scale so they can rate and record pain at different times of day, with various activities, and in response to medications and other treatments. And I review with people common descriptors of different types of pain—dull, achy, sharp, stabbing, cramping, tearing or burning, shooting, tingling, and pins and needles—that provide information to doctors about possible causes and specific treatments.

Similarly, for people with congestive heart failure, measuring and monitoring daily weight and amount of ankle swelling is invaluable in adjusting diuretic doses, improving their breathing, and exercise tolerance, as well as in preventing attacks of pulmonary edema and avoiding urgent emergency department visits and hospitalizations.

During a question-and-answer period at an evening public education forum on end-of-life care in the Midwest in which the subjects of parent care and effective advocacy were raised, a woman in her mid- to late fifties made a comment.

"Dr. Byock, my mother is eighty-three years old and basically crippled with arthritis and spinal stenosis. I live with her and am her main caregiver. She lives with pain, though we control it pretty well. She is mentally bright but has difficulties with her hearing and eyesight. I go with her to see her doctors. These days, the doctor she sees most is a hematologist because she has a condition that keeps her blood counts low. Mom likes him, but he is almost always rushed and seems distracted. Often before we have a chance to ask our questions, he is gone. What should we do?"

I recited my advocacy mantra: Be informed, prepared, polite, and persistent.

I suggested that it might be good to know the names of the people in the front office, as well as the nurses in her mother's doctor's office. Being person-centered works in both directions.

"You are already informed and can come to each appointment with a log of your mother's symptoms, a current list of all the medications she is taking, along with whatever other pertinent information you want him to know. When her doctor comes in the exam or consultation room, let him know that you have a list of questions in hand that you would like him to discuss.

"On the other end of the visit, before leaving his office, at a bare minimum, you need to understand any changes that the doctor wants you and your mother to make in her medications and treatments. You should know when, where, and with whom you are to follow up. And you must know what you and your mother should do if she develops an urgent problem."

I paused and she sat down, seemingly satisfied with my answer. But I hadn't finished and felt it was important to be explicit. "If the doctor is rushed and leaves the exam room before answering these basic questions, stay put. They need the room and someone will come back to speak with you. If someone in the office gets annoyed, you needn't raise your voice. If you wish, you have my permission to blame me. Tell them Dr. Byock said it would be unsafe to leave the office before clearly understanding these basic parts of the doctor's plan for your mother's care."

A few minutes later another middle-aged woman at the forum raised her hand and in a quivering voice described a wrenching situation.

"My father is eighty-six and just had a stroke. He can't move his left side. He's been in a nursing home for about a week. Last night when I visited, he was agitated and lying in his own urine. He said he had been pushing the button but nobody came. My father is a proud man. I am at my wit's end and don't know what to do."

I gave her the same advice I had given Michelle the morning she called my cell phone in crisis. I said, "Unless and until you can be confident that your father will get the attention he deserves, don't leave him alone. Gentle and caring people work in nursing homes, but very often there are not enough of them. Hopefully, the delay in responding to your father's buzzer was a onetime problem and has already been corrected. But if not, you and your family are within your rights both to demand better care and to personally supplement basic care the nursing home does not provide."

I continued. "My recommendations are similar to those I offered the person whose mother's hematologist is always rushed: Be polite, pleasant, and persistent. Introduce yourself and learn the names of the staff. Befriend them if possible. Tell them about your father—what name he likes to be called, what he did for work, what he loves most in life—and bring in pictures of your father in his prime. Let them know you appreciate their care, and thank them for things they do to engage and pamper your father. At the same time, if they cannot meet his basic needs, stay put. Even if push comes to shove, politely hold your ground. His needs are more important than their feelings."

Collectively, as voters and agents of accountability, citizens have vital roles to play in realizing transformative changes in America's health care system. Carefully revised laws, regulations, and public policies could accomplish some important things. A change in federal law could finally dissolve Medicare and Medicaid's arbitrary requirement that people give up treatments for their disease in order to receive hospice care. (Medicaid has already dropped the requirement for children.) New laws and regulations could ensure that staffing levels for nurses and aides in hospitals, nursing homes, and assisted living facilities rise to safe levels, in accordance with existing recommendations. Public policies could address the persistent, serious deficiencies of medical education that the Institute of Medicine and other professional bodies have cited, so that we do not graduate another generation of physicians who lack basic palliative care knowledge and skills.

People through the ages have held common fundamental wishes: to live as long and as well as possible, and, eventually, to die gently. To fulfill these wishes in the third millennium, people deserve skillful help in weighing their options and making sound medical treatment decisions.

We must train doctors in the ethics and science of decision-making and the art of discernment. If we have to march, demonstrate, litigate, and legislate to demand that doctors are competent in caring for people through the end of life, so be it.

In health care today, the only constant is change. I can think of a number of treatments that in recent memory represented the experimental fringe of care but now warrant serious consideration by people with late-stage, life-limiting disease. A decade ago, it would have been surprising for a person with far advanced leukemia or liver failure or heart failure to be evaluated and "listed" for a stem cell transplant, a liver transplant, or a heart transplant. No longer. Today, people commonly ask about these procedures and tell stories of patients they have known, read about, or seen in the news who have gone through these or other extraordinary treatments and done well.

Examples are easy to find. After having a left ventricular assist device, or LVAD, implanted—what some patients have called their "artificial heart"—former vice president Dick Cheney returned to the political fray on cable news and the lecture circuit. David Crosby of Crosby, Stills and Nash, had a liver transplant in 1995 and has thrived and continued performing for years. After his liver transplant in April 2009, visionary Apple CEO Steve Jobs lived two and a half years, during which he developed the iPad and advanced models of the iPhone.

We can expect future advances in medicine to keep coming at an ever faster pace. Treatment decisions are going to get harder as the array of treatments for failing hearts, livers, kidneys, and lungs expands beyond our current imagination. Some things won't change. People are going to grasp for treatments to keep from dying. Doctors are going to offer dying patients treatments to stay alive, even if for only a little bit longer.

And so, the problems will become ever more complex.

Experts in systems and cultural change and strategic planning consultants often quote Dwight D. Eisenhower who said, "If a problem cannot be solved, enlarge it." By shifting perspective and looking at a previously intractable problem within a new context, sometimes solutions become clear.

That is what is needed here. If we see only medical problems, we will only bring medical solutions. As long as we define our social responsibility as the need for higher-quality and more efficient health systems, doctors, and medical care at the end of life, the complexity and cost of the challenge will doom us to fail.

However, if we see the problem within a larger social framework—helping people to live in safety and as well as possible as they age, care for one another, and face the natural end of their lives—we will discover approaches that are refreshingly intuitive and many more resources than we had previously imagined were available. Then, just possibly, we can fulfill our social responsibilities and meet our loftier goals.

9.

Imagining a Care-Full Society

In the quest to provide the best care possible for people who are elderly and frail, or chronically ill at any age, it is essential for Americans to fix our national and local health care systems. But doing so will not be enough. Within this sobering realization lie reasons for hope—by expanding the problem beyond health care, potential solutions finally come into view.

The tendency to professionalize basic care and social support is well intended, but insidious. It makes care for people who are old, ill, dying, and grieving much more complicated and expensive than it needs to be. That's not the worst of it. The medicalization of aging, dying, and grief ignores the innate, healthy human drive to care for one another. It erodes core cultural roles and suppresses latent caregiving skills that reside within families and communities. Even in a person's dying— *especially in a person's dying*—family and community comprise the proper context for a person's life.

Before I suggest how things can get a great deal better, allow me to relate one last hard story that illustrates how needlessly convoluted, complex, and costly care for someone in the waning phase of life can become in America today.

Late one afternoon, we were asked by the cardiology service to consult on Denis St. Pierre, an eighty-three-year-old widower and retired butcher who was hospitalized after a fall caused by low blood pressure, kidney failure, and worsening heart failure due to a calcified aortic valve in his heart. Mr. St. Pierre was a soft-spoken man with sparse white wisps of hair on his head and feet that protruded eight inches beyond the end of his hospital bed. I imagined him in his prime, as upstanding, tall, and strong as an oak. Now, as he leaned on a walker to stand, he seemed like a weather-bent willow. Mr. St. Pierre told me, "I've been going downhill for months" in describing the steady decline in his ability to care for himself. He liked his doctors but said that the help he needed at home was hard to come by.

Whenever Mr. St. Pierre developed an acute medical problem, the health care system kicked into high gear. Three times in as many months he had been brought by ambulance to the local emergency department and then transferred to our hospital with chest pain, or a fever and sudden confusion, and, most recently, a serious fall. The fall (along with a deep forehead laceration that was sutured at the local hospital's emergency department) resulted from an episode of syncope, a term for suddenly losing consciousness and collapsing. Each time an acute medical problem occurred, cost was no obstacle. Medicare paid for the ambulance trips, blood tests, EKGs, MRIs, and his cardiac catheterization.

It would have paid for him to have heart valve surgery if Mr. St. Pierre had not respectfully refused the operation. When the surgeon explained that replacing the damaged valve carried about a 5 percent risk of a serious stroke and at least a 20 percent risk of a minor, "subclinical" stroke, Mr. St. Pierre said that he'd prefer to live—and die—with the one he had.

For the past two years Medicare paid for the kidney dialysis he received three times a week at a small dialysis center twenty miles from his northern New Hampshire town. It was lifesaving treatment. In contrast, Medicare would not pay for more basic "life support," such as someone to help Mr. St. Pierre to get up and dressed each day, to bathe him a few times a week, or to prepare his meals. These things were not health care, and Medicare and insurance guidelines make clear that only health care is covered.

Medicare also didn't pay for several health services that Mr. St. Pierre needed to prevent crises. Under Medicare rules a person must be strictly homebound to receive home health services. Since Mr. St. Pierre went to church most Sundays, the senior center a few times a month, and his barber once a month, he wasn't officially homebound and didn't qualify to have a home health nurse check his blood pressure and help him keep his medications straight. He didn't qualify for hospice care either. Under Medicare rules his only terminal diagnosis was kidney failure and it was already paying for dialysis treatments for that condition. So unless or until he decided to give up life-sustaining dialysis—which meant dying within the next five to twenty days—he was on his own at home.

Laura Rollano, our team's social worker, met with Mr. St. Pierre and, with his permission, called his niece, Anna, who lived nearly four hours away, in Connecticut. Although she visited at least one weekend each month, her own job and responsibilities as a grandmother to a toddler of her single daughter made it difficult for her to be there more often. Laura also called Mr. St. Pierre's minister, the director of the senior center in his town, and a local visiting nurse service. She was able to finagle a single evaluation visit from the local home health agency to safety-check his home, looking for fall hazards, and arranged for handrails to be installed in his shower.

Still, I was frustrated with the situation. From a systems perspective, Denis St. Pierre was clearly falling through the cracks and we didn't have a net to catch him.

When he was stable and ready for discharge, once again, like three clinical teams before us during his previous hospitalizations, we sent Mr. St. Pierre home. On any given day at home he was not sick enough to warrant acute medical attention, nor was he well enough to live safely on his own. Despite our best intentions, it felt like we—not just our team, his doctors, or our hospital, but society—were effectively leaving Mr. St. Pierre to fend for himself, ensuring that he would again lurch from one costly emergency to the next. It felt wrong and nonsensical. Plenty of money was being devoted to his care, but too much was spent reactively and in the wrong places.

Denis St. Pierre's story is not merely an example of what is wrong but, more valuably, an example of how readily secondary prevention could improve quality of care and life for frail, chronically ill people, while decreasing health care costs. Secondary prevention refers to preventing complications of illness and averting crises for people in fragile health. Simple things would have made a world of difference for Mr. St. Pierre. If he had a primary care physician—or medical home—he could have received all his medical treatments consolidated under one roof. This would have helped Mr. St. Pierre with his medications and uncovered some of the daily problems he was having at home. A weekly visit by a home health nurse would have helped, too. Discovering that his blood pressure was low and that he had been getting light-headed whenever he stood up quickly would have prevented his fall, scalp laceration, and the most recent trip to the local emergency department, as well as the subsequent transfer by ambulance to our referral medical center. A local primary care doctor could have ordered an echocardiogram and made an appointment for him to see the cardiologist who comes to their town once a week. A conversation with the cardiologist or his local primary care doctor—or a consultation with the local palliative care physician—would have established that Mr. St. Pierre clearly did not want to undergo heart valve surgery. Many thousands of dollars would have been saved.

These attributes describe patient-centered care, which is a much needed, laudable focus within health care. Yet Mr. St. Pierre's situation shows that even the best health care is not enough. To provide the best possible care and support for people during the waning phases of life— effectively and affordably—we need to be *person-* and *family-*centered.

Strategic planners and consultants in business, government, and health care challenge their clients to "think outside the box." In this case, two boxes need to be dismantled. First, we must escape our fixation with diseases and health care rather than people's well-being. Second, we must get beyond seeing people solely as individuals (a.k.a. patients) and begin seeing people as individuals *within* families and communities.

Like Mr. St. Pierre, who was widowed, approximately half of all men and three-quarters of women over the age of seventy-five live alone. Yet, also like Mr. St. Pierre, most elderly individuals who live alone have relatives and good friends who care about them and can help in a variety of ways. Mr. St. Pierre's niece drove four hours at least once a month, and spent a night on his couch, to visit and help care for him. He had a minister and a congregation who were concerned about his well-being and were trying their best to help.

Until our team got involved, after a number of avoidable crises, there was no coordinated plan for taking care of Mr. St. Pierre as a person, outside of the realm of a patient. There was no locus for such planning, and even if such a plan were developed, there was no repository to hold and make it available when needed. His niece, minister, and senior center staff were each doing the best they could, and each had some insights about his needs and ideas for supporting Mr. St. Pierre in living independently. Yet they were not in contact with one another, nor were any of them in touch with his doctors. For many months his life was harder than it needed to be. A little person-centered coordination and planning would have gone a long way.

Caregiving is fundamental to human life. It can be considered a species-specific characteristic. Anthropologist Margaret Mead was once asked what she considered the earliest evidence of civilization.

She answered that it was a human thigh bone with a healed fracture that had been excavated from a fifteen-thousand-year-old site. For an early human being to have survived a broken femur, living through the months that were required for the bone to heal, the person had to have been cared for—sheltered, protected, brought food and drink. While other animals care for their young and injured, no other species is able to devote as much time and energy to caring for the most frail, ill, and dying of its members.

Today, over 61 million Americans are engaged in the timeless role of caring for an ill or disabled young or old relative. An estimated 42 million people in this country spend an average of over eighteen hours each week—fifty to one hundred hours is not rare—helping a relative dress, bath, cook meals, dispense medications, use the toilet, change dressings, manage ostomies, apply creams, and on and on. About a quarter of baby boom generation adults, who are aging themselves, are actively providing physical care or financial support for a frail parent. Caregiving often stretches over many months and years of declining health and progressive disability.

The economic value of family caregiving has been estimated at 450 billion dollars a year, which well exceeds the total of state and federal Medicaid costs of medical care and long-term residential care combined.

Traditionally, this type of informal, unpaid caregiving has been "women's work," delegated almost reflexively to wives or daughters. Since the 1990s, as more and more boomers have engaged in parent care, this pattern has begun to change. Currently, husbands and sons are shouldering about a third of caregiving responsibilities.

Caregiving in modern times extracts a toll that may rival the strain prehistoric caregivers must have endured.

Caring for someone who is physically or cognitively frail is physically and emotionally exhausting. Caregivers often feel isolated and are at high risk for depression, anxiety, and physical illness. This is particularly true when caregivers are elderly spouses who can fall, hurt their backs, or suffer heart attacks or flares of heart failure. As caregivers' quality of life falters, their own health care costs soar and their risk of dying prematurely increases. Stress among caregivers is ubiquitous. Indeed, for millions of adult children and spouses, caregiving has become a chronic condition in itself. In a four-year surveillance study of caregivers, those who reported the highest levels of emotional and physical stress had a 63 percent higher risk of dying than those who did not.

Secondary prevention therefore rightly extends to preventing crises and stress-related illnesses among caregivers.

Denis St. Pierre's care would have been easier if his wife had not died suddenly three years earlier. Mrs. St. Pierre had been an excellent cook and doted on her husband. However, she had long-standing diabetes and coronary artery disease, as well as crippling arthritis. This points out another aspect of secondary prevention.

Elderly spouses often take good care of each other and readily detect worrisome changes in each other's well-being, which often helps prevent problems from becoming crises. With sufficient social and professional support for both individuals, cohabitating couples surely represent the most common and efficient model of home-based elder care. However, without adequate support, the stress and strain of caring can result in two people (both Medicare enrollees) being at risk of acute health problems and costly hospitalizations. It is a common situation. When one or the other member of a frail couple teeters or falls, both suffer the impact. A family-centered plan would include a way of monitoring both individuals' well-being or distress and contingency plans for intervening and shoring up support when either one teetered, hopefully before a proverbial (or actual) fall.

Because people are inextricably interconnected, when either the "patient" or the person giving care is distressed, the other suffers. Thankfully, the converse is also true: when either the patient or caregiver is well-supported and feels confident, the other benefits as well.

Caregiving will never be easy; however, simple modes of support can go a long way toward easing the stress and strain family caregivers experience. A good working relationship with the doctor and health care team of the person being cared for is probably the single most important thing that caregivers need. When caring for an ill relative or close friend, confidence is a powerful antidote to stress. Not knowing what to expect, what to do, or who to call if an emergency occurs contributes to chronic anxiety and depression among caregivers. In contrast, when caregivers feel prepared, when they know what to do and what to expect, anxiety diminishes. Good communication with professionals is reliably associated with lower levels of strain. So are coordination and continuity of care.

Some caregivers derive value from support groups of people who are dealing with similar practical and personal challenges. At our medical center, phone-based peer support groups are becoming popular as distance and the ongoing demands of caregiving make it difficult to attend meetings. A profusion of Internet-based groups and blogs have emerged as sources of information, fellowship, and support for caregivers. Although not as personal as a meeting over refreshments or even by phone, Internet-based groups offer people of diverse faiths and ethnic backgrounds a place to connect with others with similar cultural values and worldviews.

Opportunities abound to improve caregiver support and save money. Individual phone-based counseling with a nurse or social worker can support family members in problem-solving and coping with their own emotional stress without caregivers having to leave home. And without over-medicalizing the lives of the people they serve, clinicians and other helping professionals can help elders stay in their homes, safely and securely. Home health nurses especially are often a godsend for chronically ill patients and their caregivers. There are not nearly enough of them! Medicare has made it increasingly difficult for patients to qualify for home health services. In contrast, several forward-thinking insurance plans and health systems employ skilled nurses to proactively assess and manage people's chronic health problems in their home. The nurses check vital signs and weight and review patient-caregiver logs of meals, medications, and blood sugars. They explain complicated medication regimens, often catch medication errors before they occur, and prevent crises that cause suffering and result in costly hospitalizations.

Health systems that most actively utilize home services tend to be ones that are paid to take care of all their members' medical needs, rather than billing and being reimbursed piecemeal. Examples include staff-model health maintenance organizations, like Kaiser Permanente, and the Veterans Administration's Home Based Primary Care programs. These systems can readily afford to be forward thinking because they already have a financial stake in their enrolled members' care. Although these health plans are still confined to delivering *bona fide* health services, their constraints are fewer than fee-for-service insurance, Medicare, or Medicaid. Doing the right things to improve members' health and prevent crises makes obvious financial sense.

In some communities and health systems, nurses and social workers serve as case managers or health care advocates. In the past two decades, case managers have developed into a distinct profession. Professional case managers can be based in private practices, in health insurance companies and health maintenance organizations, or in social service agencies. Their roles vary but typically include helping people navigate confusing mazes of health care and social service systems. They often identify important unmet needs that can result in physical (e.g., medical) problems and preventable calamities. The best case managers advocate for their clients, facilitating access to health and social services, coordinating care, and making sure that pertinent information is reliably communicated to the doctors, other helping professionals, and service agencies who are involved in the person's care.

Because people are interconnected, the best care for seriously ill patients is also the best care for their caregiving husbands and wives. Hospice is acknowledged to represent optimal care for dying patients, improving their quality of life, and, for some, helping them live longer. It turns out that hospice may have similar benefits for caregiving spouses. In analyzing years of Medicare data on husband-wife pairs, Dr. Nicholas Christakis and associates found that even a small "dose" of hospice care—a few days of care before death—was associated with a decrease in caregivers' risks of depression after their spouse's deaths. More surprising, they also found that being a patient served by a hospice program for even a few days before death decreased the risk of a widow or widower dying prematurely. Very likely hospice care allows spousal caregivers to feel better prepared for their loved one's care and dying.

Caregiving is an inherently difficult part of life, but it is not only a burden. Remarkably, in public surveys and interviews with caregivers, despite the strain, people also commonly report gaining personal value from caring for someone they love. Since an inherent drive to provide care seems to be embedded in our genetic code, it should not be surprising that caregiving can also be deeply satisfying.

In his disturbingly insightful, yet hopeful, book *The Careless Society: Community and Its Counterfeits*, sociologist John McKnight pointedly made the case that progressive professionalization of normal life caused an erosion of natural, vital community responses to people who are ill, impoverished, or otherwise in need. In McKnight's view, doctors, psychologists, bureaucrats, and counselors are called on all too often to manage problems—through fee-based or tax-supported services— that people have been dealing with in families and communities for millennia.

Society's intentions have been good, but the outcomes have left much to be desired. Here's one example: Assisted living and skilled nursing facilities are inspected to ensure they meet standards, including that the staff are properly certified. All good. However, the emphasis on safety and privacy leads many residents of long-term care facilities to say they feel isolated. Their visitors have to be "buzzed in." They don't know their mail carrier because she leaves their mail at the front desk. Salesmen do not bother them, but Girl Scouts do not knock on the door to sell cookies, nor do trick-or-treaters at Halloween. Natural interactions with neighbors or family members of other residents are polite but superficial out of mutual respect for people's privacy.

Something is amiss when out of concerns about legal liability, volunteers at a senior center or church are told they can no longer give elders a ride in their car to an outing, the supermarket, or a doctor's appointment, barber, or beauty parlor. When a town's paid (certified and insured) transportation service is chronically understaffed, late, and unreliable, it is no mystery that frail elders are more likely to stay home and feel shut in and out of touch with their community.

Our society and culture's approach to illness, caregiving, and the end of life needs to be enlarged, old assumptions challenged, and the threads of community and professional services interwoven. We have to stop seeing illness—including terminal illness—and caregiving only as problems, and recognize them as inevitable and integral parts of a long and full life. When we do, new doors will open and more resources become visible than usually meet the eye.

A decade of gerontology research confirms what most of us instinctively knew: social connections are often as important as medical treatment in preventing physical, mental, and functional decline. Mental and physical exercise, gardening, and pets delay the progression of memory loss among many older adults and work as well as drugs in alleviating depression. Programs that pair frail elders with schoolchildren have been shown to enrich the lives of young and old.

Unpaid community volunteers are priceless resources to support frail individuals and their families, but priceless is not the same as free. To succeed, volunteer programs require infrastructure and usually paid staff. The returns on investments are high.

Years ago, I learned about a program in Wilbur, Nebraska, called Telecare, which began out of concerns over the high rate of depression among rural elders who lived alone. Telecare paired schoolchildren with older adults living alone. Each morning the kids made a brief phone call to check on their older friend. The program succeeded in enriching the lives at both ends of the phone. Although it was remarkably effective, unfortunately the program succumbed to budget cuts in the Great Recession. Yet the idea is simple to adopt and adapt. In fact, a number of RUOK programs around the country regularly check in on elders to make sure they can get to a phone. RUOK comes from "Are You OK?" In the process, relationships form between people at both ends of the phone line. It's as simple as that, but these brief, regular interactions let people who live alone know that they matter to others.

Some programs have thought outside the usual boxes and placed child day care facilities within eldercare residential facilities in which their parents work or their grandparents reside. In hundreds of hospitals across the country, foster grandparents devote time holding and rocking premature infants or newborns who are withdrawing from narcotics, methamphetamines, or crack cocaine that their mothers used during their pregnancy. Others spend time gently mentoring young children with special needs. It is not always clear who benefits more, the youngsters or oldsters.

In a few dozen communities scattered across the country, programs called Triad have teamed law enforcement agencies with aging services, elder advocates, and volunteer service groups, including youth groups such as the Key Club. The purpose of Triad is to protect elders, particularly those who live alone, from crimes and other dangers. So Triad teams perform home security and safety inspections and basic safety improvements. They enroll people in Neighborhood Watch programs and sponsor "adopt-a-senior" visits for shut-in elders and conduct safe grocery shopping trips in high-crime areas. Some Triad programs train seniors to handle telephone solicitations and door-to-door salesmen, and provide refrigerator magnet File of Life cards with critical emergency medical information and contacts.

Enlightened collaborations and pilot projects are not merely inspirational; they also demonstrate what is possible. In so doing, they help answer the strategic planning question, "What would success look like?" The challenge, nationally, lies in bringing community programs of these sorts together and sustaining them over time. Still, it is useful to imagine the fruits of a coordinated effort among community-based and professional services.

In a care-full society, a frail elder who lives alone—let's call him "Pierre St. Denis"—would receive person-centered care and community support that would include reliable transportation from his home to the local senior center once a week.

There, each Thursday from 11:00 a.m. to 1:30 p.m, our hypothetical Pierre enjoys hot lunches and listens to noontime presentations about topics ranging from practical tips for weatherizing his home and staying warm without raising heating bills, to Internet and e-mail basics, to a panel discussion on advance directives. In addition to the useful information, Pierre enjoys seeing old friends and making new ones among people his age.

The Meals On Wheels delivery staff check with him once a week to see if he had any requests or problems with his daily meals; in the process they make sure that his heat is working and that he is able to get up and around at home. A nurse from his congregation visits twice a month and has taught him to take and keep a running log of his own blood pressure. She's also taught him how to read the labels on soup cans to find the ones with lower sodium. Together they've identified and removed throw rugs and piles of newspapers and magazines from his floor that were fall hazards. One local service club installed handrails in his bathroom tub; another regularly shovels his front walk after it snows. Pierre St. Denis's community may seem utopian—nearly a mirror image of Denis St. Pierre's—but right now one or more components of this vision are in place in communities across America.

In terms of public health and public finances, secondary prevention of this sort is decidedly cost-effective. For a caring society, investments in social support and basic health surveillance for frail elders pay high rates of return through avoiding emergencies, hospitalizations, and preventable complications.

This extent of checking in and checking up on a person like Mr. St. Pierre may seem excessive to some people, perhaps a transgression of people's privacy or professional boundaries. However, the level of personal and communal interactions is typical of many societies and cultures, including American society in earlier times. Rather, our current level of privacy is peculiar to recent times and Western culture. Checking up and checking in on one another are what people in normal, caring communities do.

Too often the exaggerated emphasis on privacy in today's culture results in people not visiting others, even though they feel an urge to do so. I hear people say, "I didn't want to intrude," when the visit or call would simply have been the natural thing to do. Proper respect for people's privacy does not preclude a friend or neighbor calling or stopping by to see how another person is getting along. To state the obvious: It is morally and legally okay to show genuine concern for other people.

Just as society provides orphanages or foster care for babies without parents or relatives to care for them, so, too, our human community must recognize our most basic responsibility to care for people through the end of life.

Examples of innovative community-based programs and models for supported living abound. Here are some of my favorites. Each deserves to be developed on a far larger scale.

Naturally Occurring Retirement Communities

For people who are able to live independently and want to age in place, naturally occurring retirement communities (or NORCs) offer attractive alternatives to assisted living. NORCs are intentional communities, sometimes called villages, in which neighbors come together to share resources and help one another with basic tasks. Building from the early example of Boston's Beacon Hill Village, members pay dues, typically $350 to $1,000 annually, for help with an array of household chores like grocery shopping, shoveling snow, transportation, and fixing things. Some services are bartered or banked—one member helps prepare a holiday meal for out-of-town guests, while another helps fill out Medicare forms, and another does minor plumbing. Well over one hundred such communities exist and more are forming. NORCs are not housing projects or government programs. However, several local and state governments, most notably New York State, have supported early development of similar self-help communities. Congress included provisions to encourage the formation of NORCs in the 2006 Older Americans Act.

Program of All-Inclusive Care for the Elderly

PACE, the aptly named Program of All-Inclusive Care for the Elderly, melds medical care with a caring environment that attends to frail elders' living arrangements, their daily activities, social relations, and overall quality of life. PACE started with On Lok, a remarkable living and professional caregiving program in San Francisco for supporting frail elders. The program focused on the most vulnerable older adults, those who are unable to care for themselves and financially unable to hire the help they need on a daily basis. People served by On Lok thrived with the comprehensive, coordinated support and engagement in the community that the program provided.

Each PACE site is uniquely adapted to the locale and population it serves, yet each program amalgamates medical care with highly individualized home health and community-based services: home health care, Meals On Wheels, physical therapy, assisted living, readily accessible transportation, senior center services, group activities, and exercise groups. People love the support and sense of community they derive from PACE. So do their families.

Many PACE sites focus on people who are medically impoverished and unable to live independently at home. It is a proactive approach, with heavy emphasis on individualized assessments and ongoing problem prevention. PACE services are expensive. However, the savings to Medicare and Medicaid exceed the costs. This is particularly true since PACE not only prevents hospitalizations but PACE services are often a person's only alternative to long-term nursing home care.

Alternative Models of Long-term Care

The Eden Alternative was the brainchild of Dr. Bill Thomas, a geriatrician who proudly describes himself as "a nursing home abolitionist." Dr. Thomas identified isolation, loneliness, and boredom as factors that make residents of many nursing homes feel that life is not worth living. In Eden nursing homes and the six-to-ten-person Green House residences Thomas subsequently developed and has promulgated, there are plenty of paid staff to spend time with each resident. Plants, pets, and children are a natural part of life in these small communities. And everyone in an Eden or Green House facility—from the residents to nursing aides to the directors and administrators—has a voice in decisions that affect communal life.

This is more than idealism. It is the sort of strategic change that transforms an institution into a community. By giving residents, nursing aides, housekeepers, and cooks a say in decisions, Dr. Thomas's models foster a sense of ownership among everyone involved. Part of the return on investment here comes in forms of creativity and energy. People willingly contribute to things they own. If you are familiar with traditional nursing homes, what strikes you in walking into an Eden facility or Green House is that the place is alive! There are sounds: birds chirping or music playing with people singing, and sometimes groups of children laughing. Instead of medicinal odors, you are likely to smell freshly baked bread or cookies. Inevitably, not everyone in these facilities is having a good day every day. People are there because they are ill, senile, or otherwise frail. Still, as long-term care facilities go, the mood is remarkably bright and, somehow, more natural.

Similar initiatives include Wellspring long-term care facilities and the Pioneer Network. Importantly, these efforts concurrently strive to improve quality of care and the quality of the workplace and work life for the homes' nurses, aides, and support personnel. Experience shows that they are overwhelmingly well accepted by residents and staff.

Despite higher levels of staffing, offsetting savings make these approaches cost-effective. Savings accrue through fewer emergency hospitalizations and dramatically lower turnover among employees. So far, Eden Alternative, Green House, Wellspring, and Pioneer Network facilities are still considered "alternative" to the large majority of nursing homes, but they are gradually taking root and blossoming here and there across the country.

It would be easier to describe how to deliver the best care if there were one model or brand of systems that worked. Instead, happily, there are many.

Consider the hypothetical stories of three aging siblings: On Long Island a seventy-five-year-old man with diabetes, low vision, and early Parkinson's has his care and social services coordinated by a case manager employed by the Jewish Family and Children's Service. Across the country, his seventy-one-year-old brother, who has heart failure, atrial fibrillation, prostate cancer, and a colostomy after successful colon cancer surgery, receives care in his senior housing apartment through a PACE program in San Francisco. Their baby brother, who is just sixty-nine, has chronic lymphocytic leukemia, emphysema, and diabetes, and sees a family physician who works within a medical home that is part of Group Health in Seattle.

These brothers are served by different models of service delivery, but in each case their care is coordinated, medically up-to-date, and focused on their well-being, not just their diagnoses.

As a nation and as states and local communities, we do need revised laws and regulations and new investments in our social infrastructure of care. But those changes are merely instrumental. The bigger challenge we face is not regulatory or statutory, but cultural. Caring well for people through the end of life will require nothing less than a genuine social and cultural transformation. Simply put, it is time for our culture to grow the rest of the way up.

Our challenge is to understand illness, caregiving, death, and grief as inherently difficult, often turbulent, but entirely normal stages of life. Society, including medical and other professionals, can assist in many ways, but the need for help must not pathologize or medicalize people's experiences.

This is a lofty vision, but if our culture could mature in this way, a range of social and policy ramifications would naturally follow and we would find that solutions are neither as complicated nor as costly as many fear.

By connecting the dots among social services, community services, health care, and even basic civic services in authentically person-centered ways, we can achieve real reform and substantial cost savings. By expanding the problem, previously daunting, seemingly insolvable social responsibilities become approachable, affordable, and life-affirming.

Examples of communities in the act of caring can shine a light on the way forward. Three stories from northern New England, where I live and practice, represent for me ways that communities can grow and local cultures mature.

English professor Philip Simmons wrote about his life with ALS, also know as Lou Gehrig's disease, in *Learning to Fall*. During the last year of his life the NPR radio program *All Things Considered* ran a series of stories about how Simmons and his family were coping with his illness. When he died in July 2002 at his home in Center Sandwich, New Hampshire, NPR posted this quote from Simmons on its website: "It takes a village to care for me," he said, referring to a group called FOPAK, short for Friends of Phil and Kathryn, which had supported them during his illness. "To see a group like this working as well as it does, and to see a community as healthy as this one is, I would hope, would cause people to reflect on the possibilities that are there in their own communities. Because this can be done. Community is possible. Relationship is possible. It's up to us to create it."

Reflecting a similar experience, in December 2006, after my patient and friend Nancy Nye died, her husband, Richard Schramm, and daughter, Hope Nye Yeager, sent this note of gratitude to the members of the North Universalist Chapel Society in Woodstock, Vermont:

> We and our families would like to thank the community for all its support for Nancy Nye and us over the past two years. We have felt cradled in the hands of this community in a way that is virtually indescribable. This is our humble effort to convey to you all the many good things that you have done for us. We're sure we have missed some but this will give you a flavor of what Nancy and we experienced. There are so many people involved we will not mention any specific names. This is a thank you to the entire community.

> This community:

> Created a quilt with 99 messages of love and support

> Provided soups, salads, casseroles, desserts

> Brought meals to us and us to meals

> Wrote notes, cards, and e-mails, left phone messages, sent flowers

Helped us with second opinions, medical contacts, sorting out options, special remedies

Put our gardens to bed, stacked our firewood, cleaned our garage

Loaned us CDs and videos, meditation tapes, books

Led us in yoga classes, took us on walks

Had a meditation group with Nancy at our house

Joined us at the doctor's office and infusion rooms

Visited at the perfect times

Offered childcare, cleaning, places to escape to

Organized meals, visits, researched all kinds of things

Led a Star Island healing ceremony

Gave us a gift of Star Island souvenir photos

Gave us toys and gifts for forrest, free tickets to Billings Farm

Loaned us a juicer, body pillow, baby monitor, toys

Came and sang to Nancy at home

Stood together here in silent respect for Nancy at the beginning; cheered together after her successful first year; and hugged and cried together with her when she neared the end

Were greeters, food servers, music providers, flower organizers, video recorders, and speakers at the memorial service

Came to that service to grieve and to celebrate Nancy's life with us

For all these things and more, our family will be forever grateful. This is truly a caring community.

Hervey Durocher had retired in his late fifties from a successful career in accounting to follow his love of farming. He was sixty-nine and suffering with advanced pancreatic cancer. When I met him, he had been hospitalized for a bile duct infection, which, fortunately, had rapidly responded to IV antibiotics. His oncologist asked our team to help Hervey and his wife, Joan, in clarifying their goals for care. When we discussed his goals, Hervey was emphatic. "I just want to get back up on my tractor," he said. It was his way of saying, "I just want to go home."

Joan assured us that they could manage at home and that there would be plenty of help from family, friends, and neighbors. She proudly described her husband as a strong, gentle man who was always ready to help others. That afternoon, I spoke with their family physician, Dr. Donald McDonah, who happens to be the medical director of the hospice program in their rural southern New Hampshire community. Dr. McDonah and I coordinated plans for home hospice care.

The next day, we discharged Mr. Durocher. Hervey died peacefully in their family's home a couple of weeks later.

One afternoon about a month after Mr. Durocher's death, I received a letter from Joan with a card from his memorial service and a request that I give her a call. When we spoke by phone, Joan described the funeral at the local Congregational church. She told me that as the funeral procession wended its way through the rural country roads from their church to the cemetery, past fields and saltbox farmhouses, every farm had its tractors turned to the road with their headlights blazing in silent memorial for Hervey.

In their grief and the love for a friend they had lost, this community of men and women from varied backgrounds, faiths, and political beliefs stood together on common ground.

When people are engaged in communities, friends and neighbors tend to rise to their and their families' needs. One might chalk it up to adversity bringing out the best in people. There's truth in that. But what I have witnessed again and again is deeper and more profound than kindness. It is the natural, uncontrived, and unconstrained way that people living *in community*—rather than merely *in proximity*—respond to one another. In healthy human communities, it would seem odd to do anything less.

10.

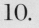

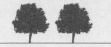

Standing on Common High Ground

In one sense, the real reason that thousands upon thousands of Americans still die badly is that we collectively allow it to happen. Of course, no one votes to make people suffer. But as a society and body politic we tolerate widespread, needless suffering among seriously ill people and their families and well-documented deficiencies in medical care and social systems.

Our inaction on this crisis of public health is incongruent with our character as a society and culture. We are a caring and generally sensible people. Despite our culturally ingrained avoidance of the topics, in my clinical experience, when push comes to shove, individuals and families move beyond their resistance to talk seriously about how they or the person they love should be cared for through the end of life. Yet collectively, despite overwhelming evidence of pervasive problems, we act as if push hasn't come to shove.

Instead, an amalgam of politics and religion has made dying and end-of-life care culturally toxic. Political correctness and an overt desire to avoid conflict stifle substantive dialogue and debate. Yet open discussion that encompasses medical and social perspectives, including multicultural ethnic and religious worldviews, is exactly what is needed. With issues this big, diverse social dialogue and debate, even if heated, are essential for developing constructive public policies and large-scale corrective actions.

Mortality should be the one thing that brings all people together. In science fiction, when a planet-killing asteroid is headed toward Earth, people set petty differences aside. Historically, in the face of major natural disasters, even differences between bitter enemies can suddenly look pretty small. Death is the natural disaster that awaits us all. Instead of bringing people together in a common purpose, how we die has become a polarizing subject, rife with acrimony and righteous indignation. The irony would be funny if the social paralysis it caused were not so damaging.

Unfortunately, in many people's minds and in the media, the question of whether or not to legalize physician-assisted suicide has become a proxy for how we die. It is a matter most audibly and visibly debated in America's legislatures and courts. Both settings tend to dichotomize each matter considered and impose an adversarial framework to any discussion. Legislators can either vote for or against a bill. The court can either find for or against a plaintiff. Creative solutions are all but foreclosed.

In these adversarial arenas, the fight over physician-assisted suicide makes it appear as if a cultural chasm divides Americans. In fact, the chasm is a mirage, an artifact of the boxing rings to which our social discourse has been confined. The differences of values and opinions over physician-assisted suicide are real and deserve to be debated. But this one issue is a poor proxy for the subjects of how we die and how we can best care for people through the end of life. Our differences are dwarfed by the common high ground of values, shared wishes for care, and goodwill toward one another on which we all stand. It is on this common ground that we can build better systems of medical care and social support and realize our full social potential.

I was once a combatant in this fight. From the early 1980s through the early 1990s, I was active in opposing legalizing physician-assisted suicide. Although I continue to believe it is ill-advised public policy, years ago I realized that the debate itself is destructive and so became a noncombatant. For me the most socially damaging aspect of the assisted suicide debate is its power to conscript all the legislative energy and editorial page attention (both priceless and limited commodities) that might actually resolve the sorry state of dying in America. The debate is a brawl on the lawn of a burning building. The people trapped inside are suffering and pleading for help, while would-be rescuers and passersby stand captivated by the fistfight. With each round of legal wrangling, each side hopes to score a knockout. Meanwhile, the volume of the melee effectively drowns out any substantive, constructive discussion.

Ironically, in the midst of what at times seems like a hopelessly polarized electorate, conditions are ripe for constructive policies. Despite different political persuasions, most Republicans and Democrats have similar views on whether individuals have the right to make their own decisions about end-of-life medical care. According to Pew Research Center data, equally strong majorities of both major political parties, as well as Independents, approve of laws that let patients decide about being kept alive through medical treatment. In Pew surveys only 22 percent of people felt that doctors must always try to save or prolong life, while 70 percent felt that patients should sometimes be allowed to die.

New Hampshire is a hotbed of politics, but even here the common ground of values on which we stand is palpable. Because of the Granite State's first-in-the-nation presidential primary, New Hampshire citizens take seriously their responsibility for vetting would-be presidential candidates—and winnowing the field. This is especially evident during elections in which there is no incumbent president. Presidential hopefuls come to nearly every town and, it sometimes seems, every street corner of the state. It is retail politics at its best. If you wish, it is easy to meet and ask candidates—one of whom will soon be president—direct questions.

In the spring of 2007, with fiercely contested Republican and Democratic primaries and health care reform high on the list of issues on voters' minds, colleagues and I from Dartmouth-Hitchcock Medical Center convened eight citizen forums throughout New Hampshire. We met early evenings, at senior centers, churches, and Elks lodges, from Littleton to Keene to Concord to Portsmouth. A total of 463 citizens spent over two hours in discussion and, through participant-response keypads, answered detailed questions about what was most important to them and for the people they love during "the waning phase of life." We also asked participants what they wanted the presidential candidates to know as they developed health and social policies to improve the lives of frail elders, people with serious illness, and their family caregivers.

The results showed a striking degree of agreement with ideas and policy proposals that have been put forward by various governmental panels, professional associations, and patient organizations. More than 80 percent of participants at these community forums indicated it was very important or extremely important to have their dignity respected, preferences honored, pain controlled, and not to leave family with debt. Only 7 percent felt it was very important or extremely important to be kept alive as long as possible. The large majority wanted to be at home at the end of life, only 1 percent said they would prefer being in a hospital, and not a single participant wanted to be in a nursing home at the end of life.

Participants wanted hospice and palliative care to become routine: 94 percent favored mandating coverage for adult and children's hospice and palliative care through all private insurers, state Medicaid, and state employee-based coverage. Over 80 percent favored removing Medicare requirements of a six-month-or-less life expectancy and being willing to give up disease treatments in order to receive hospice care. Ninety-three percent favored making residential hospice available when needed; fully 60 percent felt that doing so was extremely important.

They wanted doctors and nurses to be well trained and skilled in care of elders and dying people: 97 percent felt that medical and nursing students must be taught basic knowledge and skills required to care for older adults and people with chronic illness. Similarly, 97 percent agreed that the faculty of medicine and nursing schools should be required to have knowledge and skill in geriatrics, palliative, and end-of-life care. Ninety-four percent would require medicine and nursing schools to teach the health effects of caregiving and support for family caregivers. Over 90 percent felt strongly that physicians should be required to pass tests in basic pain management and end-of-life care in order to obtain licenses to practice and prescribe medications.

The results showed marked differences of opinions on only two subjects, hastening death and prayer. Asked to rate the importance of "having assisted suicide available if I am suffering," 40 percent of participants felt that it was very important or extremely important, while 39 percent rated it "not at all" important. Similarly, "having an injection to cause death (euthanasia) available if I am suffering" was rated very important or extremely important by 34 percent, while 40 percent felt that it was not important at all. A minority felt that being prayed with (44 percent) or being prayed for (41 percent) was very or extremely important, while 24 and 23 percent, respectively, felt prayer was not important at all.

These 463 New Hampshirites hardly comprise a representative sample of America. They were mostly white (reflecting the overwhelmingly Caucasian makeup of the state's population), middle-aged or older. Three-fourths were women. The group was well educated, with 70 percent having a bachelor's or graduate degree. But one can say with confidence that this group was comprised of likely voters—primary voters—people whose opinions matter to politicians. And the results show that the extent of common ground dwarfs the differences of partisan politics.

The toxicity of the assisted suicide debate has spilled over and threatens to poison important public discussions about how we can most wisely use finite resources to provide the best care for the greatest number of people. "Rationing health care" is the now familiar, albeit incendiary, shorthand that the "Pro-life" activists have successfully assigned to this vital subject. Through the filter of the culture war, opposing camps are characterized as secular humanists who want to limit lifesaving treatments to people who are no longer productive versus God-fearing religious conservatives who believe every life has value and only God can make decisions of life and death. As in all wars, the opponents see things very differently and don't like one another. They are much more likely to aim invectives than to actually speak with one another. This is no way for our caring society to deal with a very real problem that *we already have.*

In the most basic, unvarnished terms the situation is this: human beings inhabit a planet that is merely 24,901.55 miles (40,075.16 kilometers) in circumference, less distance than many people drive each year. We hurtle through deep space, held on the surface of this green Earth by an invisible force of gravity, protected from the frigid galactic void by a thin blanket of air. The fundamental question that confronts us all is: *How then shall we live?*

I do not consider myself a religious person. I do not regularly attend religious services or belong to a congregation, and so, in the simplistic dichotomy of the rationing debate, I probably fit the secular humanist description. However, my answer to the question *How then shall we live?* is rooted in my Jewish upbringing and my experience of Judaism.

Within the worldview in which I was raised, the primal social compact is not a contract; it is a covenant. Human beings belong to one another before we are born and long after we die. In a morally healthy society, people are born into the welcoming arms of the human community and die from the reluctant arms of community. Within this covenantal experience, the well-being of others affects my own quality of life.

On this small planet, even in our wealthy country, we have finite resources. Our challenge as a moral people is to use those resources wisely, justly, and humanely.

Even if the United States could absorb rising health care costs that are on track to exceed 20 percent of our gross domestic product, some vital assets would remain limited. The clearest example is donor organs for transplantation. Implantable artificial hearts and other organs are on the distant horizon. For the foreseeable future, many more people will need a donor heart, liver, or lung to survive than will be able to get them. Life-and-death decisions such as these will continue to challenge our society and culture. We all have a stake in how such decisions are made.

TAKING THE LONG VIEW, we are still a young civilization and our culture is a work in progress. In our policies, programs, and plans for caring for people through the end of life, we have been acting childishly: ignoring basic responsibilities, indulging in magical thinking (*If we ignore it, maybe it will go away*), and fighting without regard to the consequences.

As a society and culture, it is time to set aside childish ways and act like adults.

Yes, someday we are each going to die! Let's get over it—so that we can get on with seriously addressing the question, *How shall we live?* to the fullest extent.

Each ethnic and each religious tradition will answer the question of how people live and care for one another through the end of life in ways that are consistent with the tradition's distinct vision for responsible and full lives as individuals and families.

As a nation, our collective cultural vision of the best care possible for people through the end of life will comprise a diverse and colorful tapestry of experiences that individuals and communities deem desirable.

Health care, particularly my own field of hospice and palliative care, must contribute panels to that tapestry in the form of stories of people who were comfortable, for whom systems worked, and experiences of people who felt well within themselves and as a family through the final days of life. Projects that deliberately collect and curate stories can contribute first-person accounts. StoryCorps, founded by David Isay, is a nonprofit organization that has traveled the country collecting interviews between pairs of people, in each case relatives or close friends, about what they consider to be the most meaningful memories of their relationship and shared history. StoryCorps' Legacy Initiative (of which I am an adviser) is extending this process to people who are facing the end of life. All of StoryCorps' interviews are archived at the Library of Congress and a selected few are broadcast on public radio. In this manner, narrative histories, photos, and graphic images can weave a multitextured cultural fabric of dying and caregiving experiences that will hopefully expand our collective vision of what is possible, and raise our expectations and aspirations.

The medical profession, along with nursing and the other health care professions, have important roles to play in keeping our national discourse grounded in the fundamental social responsibility to care well for the most ill and frail of our members. It is clearly medicine's job to set and enforce high standards for physician practice and training. Medicine also has a legitimate role—one among many of society's professions—in fostering cultural maturation with regard to how we live through illness, caregiving, dying, and mourning. But as I've argued, questions of how we die, how we care for one another, and how we grieve are only partially the domain of medicine. Full consideration of these fundamental questions extends beyond the domain of health care. Social standards of care and support, allocation of resources, and the ethics of decision-making must be developed in collaboration with the professions of ministry, sociology, law, and ethics.

This brings us back to the issue of physician-assisted suicide. In discharging its responsibility to society as a repository of special knowledge and expertise, the profession of medicine as a whole, and the specialty of hospice and palliative care in particular, officially oppose hastening death.

In fact, a formal ethical principle and precept of palliative care holds that the practice of palliative care does not intentionally hasten death. While not purposefully political, this tenet has deliberate cultural significance and, therefore, inevitable political implications.

The founders of the discipline understood that the key distinction—between letting terminally ill people die and intentionally ending their lives—was essential to maintain public trust in the doctors and nurses who work in hospice and palliative care. The wisdom of explicitly distinguishing *caring* for people from *causing people's death* is evident in our present times. Today, distrust of doctors is at an all-time high and some accuse hospice and palliative care clinicians of promoting a "culture of death" when we allow dying people to leave this life gently, without subjecting them to CPR or mechanical ventilation or dialysis or medical nutrition.

The predominant opposition to hastening death, among doctors and other clinicians, is not primarily religious, at least not for most. It is, however, rooted in profound respect for life that clinicians share with many theologians, clerics, and religious people.

In November 1996, Joseph Cardinal Bernardin, archbishop of Chicago, wrote to the United States Supreme Court as justices were considering the landmark physician-assisted suicide case of *Vacco v. Quill*. He wrote as a cleric, but also as someone living with—and dying from—pancreatic cancer.

I am at the end of my earthly life. There is much that I have contemplated these last few months of my illness, but as one who is dying I have especially come to appreciate the gift of life. I know from my own experience that patients often face difficult and deeply personal decisions about their care. However, I also know that even a person who decides to forgo treatment does not necessarily choose death. Rather, he chooses life without the burden of disproportionate medical intervention.

Bernardin's perspective powerfully articulates the stance of secular hospice and palliative care. It is not about Catholicism or religion, but about respecting and honoring all of life.

Words matter and both sides in the assisted suicide debate have forcibly expropriated important terms—"dignity" and "Pro-life"—by branding them. Once branded the terms take on new, proprietary meanings. The linguistic contortions and etymological twists result in complicating (at best) and distorting (more commonly) social discussions of how we should regard and can best care for people who are nearing the end of life. These linguistic contortions have social consequences beyond merely ignoring the actual etymology of the terms.

Proponents of legalizing physician-assisted suicide have branded "death with dignity" in a way that implies that people who are dying are not already dignified. But, of course, they are. Indeed, the preamble to the UN's 1948 Universal Declaration of Human Rights states that "recognition of the inherent dignity and of the equal and inalienable rights of all members of the human family is the foundation of freedom, justice and peace in the world." The declaration formalizes a human value that is rooted in fundamental anthropological facts. The impulse to honor and care for our most vulnerable members—our infants, elderly, injured, and ill—is a defining trait of our species, literally part of our humanity. Most of us will be physically dependent and intimately cared for by others in the days before we die. This fact does not destine us to become undignified. It simply confirms that we are human.

At least as problematic, faith-based groups opposed to physician-assisted suicide have effectively branded the term "Pro-life." What does that make everyone else? The distortions that arise from these linguistic transgressions are far-reaching.

It is not a political statement to observe that doctors are inherently Pro-life. Their roles and responsibilities require it. (The same is true for nurses.) As patients—and as citizens—we want our pediatricians, family doctors, internists, obstetricians, surgeons, emergency

care physicians, and critical care physicians to be *pro*tectors and *pro*po-
nents of life, health, and longevity. Don't we? We should worry if they
are not.

I am ardently Pro-life, but it has nothing to do with "Pro-life" politics. I am simply one of thousands of doctors and nurses who work in our
nation's emergency departments, ICUs, cancer centers. Collectively, we
represent the most authentically Pro-life segments of American society.
The Pro-life agenda we advance is apolitical. We strive to save and preserve people's lives and care for people who go on to die. To fully and
authentically affirm life, we must affirm *all of life*, including dying, death,
and grief.

My own Jewish upbringing helped to shape my opinions and ori-
entation toward care, but the influence has far more to do with social
justice than theology.

I grew up during the 1950s and 1960s when the cultural-political current of daily headlines, nightly news, popular music, and movies lifted
voting rights, desegregation, women's rights, and the rights of children
along what seemed like a progressive arc of civilization. In my family,
those values were embraced. My parents were raised in northern New
Jersey, first- and second-generation descendants of Eastern European
Jewish immigrants. Jewish cultural values of fairness, generosity, service
to others, and the importance of community infused my upbringing far
more than prayers. The Jewishness of my upbringing revered life more
than any notion of God. Looking back, I suppose it is not surprising that
the plight of dying people would seem egregious to me—not merely a
medical deficiency, or even a lapse of ethical practice, but a tear in the
social fabric.

IT IS TIME TO REVISIT the ethics of caring for people through the end
of life from a fresh perspective. From a broad, *how-shall-we-live?* social
perspective, the analyses and guidelines of bioethics seem constricted

and incomplete. The early history of bioethics was formed by deliberations and court decisions having to do with people's right to refuse
unwanted treatments and situations under which it is acceptable to
remove life support. During an era spanning the 1970s through the mid-
1990s—a period roughly corresponding to the development of hospice and palliative care—advances in clinical ethics reflected distinctly
subtractive themes. A series of U.S. Supreme Court decisions (such as
those of Karen Ann Quinlan, Elizabeth Bouvia, and Nancy Cruzan),
consensus statements, and published guidelines by professional associations further defined when treatments can be withheld or withdrawn.
As practiced and taught, contemporary bioethics still largely concerns
under what circumstances, by what means, and to what extent individuals, patients' families, and formally named legal surrogates can decline
life-prolonging treatments (such as CPR, surgery, mechanical ventilation, and artificial nutrition and hydration). While necessary and important, such guidance is insufficient.

Surely, a moral and healthy society's response to caring for people
with advanced age or life-threatening conditions encompasses more
than a person's right to refuse medical treatments. A fuller social and
communal view of ethics would also clarify the circumstances and
extent to which people must be accorded medical care—basic preventive care, as well as extraordinary life-prolonging treatments. Even more
important, a complete ethical framework would encompass whether and
to what extent society first must meet the basic human needs that people
have as they approach life's end. Basic elements of human care underpin
how we regard and respond to others—our ethics as people become
sicker and more physically dependent:

Shelter from the elements. A caring society metaphorically says to the
frail or dying person, "We will keep you warm and dry."

Help with personal hygiene. The community reassures the person who is
too frail to care for himself or herself, "We will keep you clean."

Assistance with elimination. Family or, on behalf of society, clinicians (typically nurses or nurse aides), say, "We will help you with your bowels and bladder function."

Provision of food and drink. We can say, "We will always offer you something to eat and drink—and help you to do it."

Keeping company. Society can say to people who are dying, especially those who are "unbefriended," "We will be with you. You will not have to go through this time in your life entirely alone."

Alleviating suffering. Certainly today, society can say, "We will do whatever we can, with as much skill and expertise as available, to lessen your discomfort." Yet it is only this final element that is dependent on clinical expertise.

"COMPETENCE," "thoroughness," "continuity," and "technical expertise" are terms that describe attributes of the best care. In addition to all these qualities, the phrase "tender, loving care" has long been a *sine qua non* for excellence in human caring. This is more than a platitude. In responding to people who are facing the end of life, loving care is an authentic and invaluable clinical modality.

Love is, after all, the primal impetus and sustaining force of all the caring professions. There is nothing unethical or unseemly about loving our patients. It is worth stating explicitly that we must remain aware of the power we have over the sick and vulnerable people we serve and must be careful to avoid manipulating patients or acting for our own self-gain in any way. When those simple guidelines are followed, love in a clinical relationship is wholesome and therapeutically powerful.

Often when a physician cannot imagine what else to do for someone who is feeling helpless and hopeless—for whom life has no value—I find that love is the answer. I realize how glib and saccharine that may sound. But in practical ways, loving care opens up a full range of possibilities that are not seen through the problem-based filters of medicine. People who are ill can be accompanied, supported in completing valued tasks, and engaged in community. Even when they are fully dependent and nearing death, people can be pampered.

Love is not all we need—science, technology, good judgment, and sound policy are also required—but without love we are without hope of fixing this crisis. However, loving care is not a philosophical stance only; it has tangible therapeutic applications and effects.

Loving care represents the full expression of the ethical principle of beneficence. Loving care counterbalances subtractive themes and completes an ethical framework for clinical care. In loving care, therapeutic interventions are not bound by responding to problems and suffering; loving care extends beneficence by encompassing actions intended to elicit pleasure and joy. Several integrative or complementary therapies can contribute to patients receiving loving care.

For example, I asked Daren McCallum's parents, whom we met in chapter 5, what had helped them during the many days when he languished so close to death in the ICU. In addition to finding one critical care attending physician who would consistently answer their questions, and a nurse who showed them where to find towels and where to take a shower, Daren's mother, Marilyn, surprised me by saying that Reiki had helped her get through the long anxious days. I hadn't been aware that Reiki was being offered to families of ICU patients. Reiki is a complementary therapy that is being increasingly used throughout the medical center as a way of soothing people. A dozen or more volunteers, each of whom has completed a formal training course, see people in the cancer center, in the same-day surgery waiting room, preoperative testing area, and, I now know, the ICU.

Reiki looks like touch-less massage. The person performing Reiki holds his or her hands on or just above the surface of a person's body and, with motions of hand and arms, moves energy to or from places that hurt and places that need healing. As far as I know, Reiki has no scientific basis and is not billed for or paid. But for many people, it works. They feel better after having it and often ask to have it performed again. This may very well be the purest form of the placebo effect: one person's healing intention causing a therapeutic effect in another. All the more reason to recommend it. People love it and I have yet to hear of any dangerous side effects.

Our medical center sees nothing wrong in nurturing and pampering people when we can. Our No One Alone volunteers distribute newspapers to patients in the hospital and to people sitting in the waiting rooms of the ICU and OR (operating room), as well as the cancer center's clinics.

We have support groups for patients with cancer and their families. For a few hours each week, the center employs an artist, a creative writer, and a musician who travels with a small harp. The artist sits with people in the cancer infusion room and in the hospital to sketch or watercolor images. The writer helps people express thoughts and feelings in short poems or stories. The musician wanders through the infusion room and the inpatient cancer floor with her harp and a small folding stool and settles before a patient's recliner or bed to play for a few minutes at a time. All of this may seem trivial, but sometimes little things make a big difference in people's quality of life.

Clare Wilmot is a surgeon in her mid-fifties who was hospitalized for four months during arduous treatments for leukemia. Through two failed stem cell transplants and a series of life-threatening viral, bacterial, and fungal infections, and a third stem cell transplant that was finally successful, Clare was mostly confined to her room. After being discharged, she continues to be an outpatient and avails herself of the healing arts program in the cancer center's infusion suite.

She wrote me a note to say that as a doctor she had never realized how important the arts and music could be, but that they made her feel loved and cared for.

"Margaret's harp made me cry, where I have not cried more than once in this whole process . . . she has found music that has touched me so deeply, that I felt refreshed afterward, connected to the musicians and life. . . . Rebecca has encouraged and cajoled and taught me to paint with watercolors, so that my artist daughter was impressed. Marv came and pulled a few poems out of me and assigned homework. . . . He and I will submit poems to an International Symposium on Poetry and its place in Healing! They have all become friends and I thank you for your foresight and ability to run such a program! My symptoms are all manageable—in large part due to the creative forces you have provided."

LOVING CARE CAN HELP alleviate suffering, but a patient does not need to be suffering to benefit. Seriously ill people often benefit from being nurtured or pampered a bit.

Massage, Reiki, music, expressive arts and writing, and, perhaps, having a volunteer visit can make someone's difficult day a little lighter and brighter.

Hard-boiled cynics may scoff at my alleged naivety. Having spent nearly a decade and a half working in emergency departments—where cynicism and dark humor are as ubiquitous as dark coffee—I can understand their doubts. In this situation, however, cynicism is not warranted.

I regularly invite journalists and policy makers to spend a day with our team at Dartmouth-Hitchcock and I have seen jaded agency administrators, politicians, and journalists melt when they see loving care in action: Seeing a terminally ill patient laugh while reading the newspaper with one of our No One Alone volunteers. Glimpsing a nurse humming as she gives a debilitated patient a bed bath, as if the purpose of the act was to cause pleasure and the person became clean merely as a by-product. Witnessing a person in pain fall gently asleep while having a foot massage. Attending our morning clinical huddle and hearing us wrestle with strategies for relieving a person's pain, but also ideas for helping a family honor and celebrate a person who is facing the end of life.

A politically conservative state legislator was with our team for a day during the week we were helping to care for Mrs. Gold. When I met her, Mrs. Gold had been in the hospital for nine days and in the ICU for seven days, a victim of insidious pulmonary hypertension and pulmonary fibrosis that had caused no symptoms but had been damaging her lungs and heart for many months. Now, at age seventy-eight, she needed mechanical ventilation to breathe, but she steadfastly refused to be intubated. Instead, she was fitted with a BiPAP mask that blew oxygen-enriched, compressed air through her nose and mouth and into her lungs. She could speak in short well-planned sentences if the BiPAP was removed for a few moments, but she mostly communicated by gesturing expressively with her hands and eyes. She had no problem conveying that she was not happy. She told us in one breath, "I don't want to live like this."

We were able to make her comfortable with small doses of morphine. She was alert, not suffering, but ready to die. She had raised four daughters and two sons after her husband had died when he was just thirty-eight years old. As the matriarch of her large family, she wanted to make sure they understood and accepted her decision to die and was willing to hang on for a few days for their sake.

Her children and their spouses and her many grandchildren ached with grief at the thought of her dying. Ultimately, however, each one supported her decision. During one of several meetings with her family, a daughter in her forties spoke for her assembled relatives. "We're as close as any family could ever hope to be."

Overnight her ICU room was transformed into family space. There were at least thirty photos hung around her ICU room, including one of her own mother as a bride. She was never alone, usually there were two or more family members present. Her pastor visited her every other day.

I was present on the Saturday afternoon when the BiPAP was removed. We gave her small doses of medication (morphine and lorazepam); she was sleepy but awake. There was never a hint of distress.

The last thing Mrs. Gold saw in this world were the faces of her six children and two grandchildren, all touching a part of her, all smiling with tears in their eyes, each saying, "We love you, Mom." One said, "Tell Dad we send our love."

These sorts of gentle, loving end-of-life experiences happen fairly commonly in the homes of hospice patients. In reflecting on the case I realized that in the minds of most people, ICU treatment and hospice-like care are polar opposites, almost the antithesis of each other. Indeed, just a few years ago, I could only have dreamed of being able to extend this level of whole-person, whole-family, tender and loving care in an academic medical center's ICU. No longer. Every few months, it seems, we celebrate a wedding in the ICU or conduct a renewal of vows in the hospital's chapel. This is exceptional, but not rare. On that Saturday, I was glad that I was being "shadowed" by three second-year medical students. They stood beside me as Mrs. Gold died and witnessed what good care through the end of life looks like.

The following Monday, I called the legislator and reported how Mrs. Gold had died. He agreed that her experience was illuminating. Then he said, "That's all great, but there isn't a program like this everywhere!"

True enough. My question is, Why not?

Socially and culturally, something akin to the birthing movement is needed to transform care through the end of life. As recently as the 1960s, pregnancy and childbirth were treated as solely medical events. Many women were given general anesthesia during labor. Mothers and babies were kept in the hospital for five or more days.

Fathers were not allowed into delivery rooms. When the baby boom generation was having children, women and their husbands demanded expert medical treatment but stated clearly that pregnancy and child-birth were fundamentally personal experiences.

How things have changed! Today, natural childbirth is encouraged. Fathers are not merely allowed to be present but strongly encouraged to participate as birthing coaches and to attend birthing classes. Hospitals compete for baby business by maintaining homey birthing suites that can accommodate a couple—and family.

The specialty of obstetrics ultimately embraced these changes. The shift by organized medicine was aided by research that showed that having fathers involved was safe and a good thing for the well-being of all involved. However, this transformation was not driven by an evidence base but by strong citizen and consumer action. Without citizen-consumer pressure, these advances would likely have remained confined to pilot projects at forward-thinking institutions.

Now, it's the other end of the life cycle demanding attention. As we age, care for parents and other loved ones, and approach our own dying, the baby boom generation can wrest from medicine the quintessentially personal experience of dying, as well as caring for someone you love as they die. We are well positioned to meet the challenge. Boomers may be older, but we are still the "me generation." We still question authority—and we only accept the very best.

As we did when we were of childbearing age, it is again time to take back responsibility for the care of the people we know and love.

We all want "the best care possible" for our loved ones. It's time to determine what that means in some detail and bring citizen and consumer pressure to bear to get it. We can expect—and must insist upon—expert medical care that is consistent with the needs and preferences of our friends and loved ones. Beyond these basics, we have the capacity to care for people in ways that not only ensure relative comfort but also allow them to feel wanted, worthy, and dignified during their terminal frailty.

Hardly a radical set of expectations.

Nowadays, well-informed citizens and consumers clearly see common deficiencies in care and have begun to imagine what the best care possible looks like. In demanding the best care for themselves or someone they love, they advance needed changes for us all.

THE FEAR OF DYING BADLY should suffice to bring people of all races, religions, ethnic roots, and political persuasions together to fix this

crisis. Yet there are higher emotions, comprising the transcendent pin-
nacle of human experience, which also draw our attention to the end of
life. For all the suffering that surrounds dying and death, many people
experience such times as sacred.

THE CONFRONTATION WITH DEATH lays bare the spiritual core of the
human condition. The force of impending death acts like a hot wind
to strip away all pretenses and expose each person's elemental essence.
What we call spiritual is our innate response to the awe-inspiring and
terrifying mystery of human life and the universe. A heightened awareness of the essential mystery of life and the potential to evoke terror and
awe affects anyone who ventures close to a person's dying. Confronted
with the mystery of life—and death—we reflexively try to make some
meaning of our experience in the world, strengthen our relationships
with others, and feel part of something larger and more enduring than
ourselves.

Throughout time and across cultures, people have conveyed wisdom
for dealing with life's mysteries through religions. Anthropologists and
archaeologists have found evidence of spiritual practices throughout
human history. Religious teachings, customs, rituals, traditions, stories, and
songs have guided individuals and families through births and deaths,
celebrations and grief. Not surprisingly, people who have a deep religious faith often feel it is a source of strength and comfort in dealing
with illness, caregiving, death, and grief.

Spirituality is rightly considered the province of religion, but it is not
an exclusive province. Accompanying people who are dying has taught
me that human life is inherently spiritual, whether or not a person practices a religion.

One afternoon in clinic, I asked Mr. Grady, a gruff, wizened farmer
from Thetford, Vermont, if he considered himself a spiritual person. It is
a question I ask every patient, unless the person has already volunteered

information about his or her beliefs. I ask, because I can't count the number of times I would have surmised wrongly.

"Nah, not me," Mr. Grady said with a wry, tight smile. Congestive heart failure and lung disease gave him the habit of delivering short, considered bursts of words, all spoken in a thick New England brogue.

I probed a bit. "Do you have a sense of where we go after we leave this life?"

"Yup," he replied with a chuckle, his smile giving way to a broad, toothless grin. "The worms go in; the worms go out," he replied, his hand and wrist mimicking an undulate in motion.

I was curious about where he was planning to be buried. "Where will the worms go in and out of your bones, Mr. Grady?"

"Oh, we have a family cemetery on a hill in Thetford," his tone now earnest between pauses to breathe. "We Gradys have been buried there since the early 1800s." Another breath. "I suspect my grandchildren and their grandchildren will be there, too."

Mr. Grady didn't pray, attend church, or believe in God. However, his strongly felt connection to the land and his family, including generations of ancestors that preceded him and generations that would follow, seemed authentically spiritual to me.

Our team members—and increasingly, clinicians in our field—sometimes use poetry to explore spiritual aspects of people's experience.

Alice Fehling was a forty-seven-year old woman with advanced intraperitoneal cancer and ascites who was admitted to the hospital when her leg suddenly turned cold and blue. After the successful removal of an arterial clot restored circulation to the limb, she developed kidney failure. During rounds one Sunday morning, I visited Alice in her hospital room. Following the requisite pain and bowel update, we indulged in musings about illness, healing, God, and love. The conversation began when I asked about the collection of Rumi's poems on her bedside table. We read a few and then I shared a favorite poem and asked her to guess who wrote it.

You do not need to leave your room,
Remain sitting at your table and listen.
Do not even listen, simply wait.
Do not even wait, be quiet, still and solitary.
The world will freely offer itself to you to be unmasked.
It has no choice.
It will roll in ecstasy at your feet.

"THAT'S WONDERFUL, but I have no idea who the poet is," Alice said.

"Franz Kafka," I replied.

Alice was surprised that Kafka, the quintessential existentialist whose writing typically portrayed the universe as cold and impersonal, leaving each individual exposed to circumstance and happenstance, would offer a vision of an ecstatic world. This led Alice and me to talk about chaos theory, fractals, and patterns within randomness. She spoke about healing and well-being in the face of loss, and her sense of God within us all and all that is. She knew she was dying and hated to leave her husband with whom she felt ever more deeply in love. Alice said that except for her physical ailments, she had felt "well" and alive in these last few months.

The spiritual impact of death's approach is often felt by those who know and care for a person who is ill. Birth, illness, and death, even with the financial strain, time pressures, and turmoil in health care, imbue clinical care with a spiritual dimension.

Doctors and nurses only rarely talk to one another about these things. However, over the years many colleagues have spoken to me about accompanying patients in their final days, hours, and moments before death. Again and again, the words "privilege" and "sacred" are part of their descriptions. "There was something sacred about being there when Mrs. Jones passed." Or, "It was a sacred moment for the family," adding, "for me, too." Along with, "It was a privilege to help care for

Mrs. Jones. I feel fortunate to have been there as she died." Or simply, "What a privilege!"

My unscientific sample suggests that the experience of sacredness and privilege in the presence of these events is shared by people of all religions, politics, and temperaments. I have exchanged nods of silent recognition of the indefatigable quality of people's deaths with unsentimental surgeons and tightly wrapped intensivists. It is not just the end of life, but somehow a culmination of human experience. To those who have had the experience, no explanation is necessary; to those who have not, no explanation will be sufficient.

None of this suggests that modern clinicians harbor a religious agenda. My sense is that "sacred" is merely the word that most closely fits what many of us experience. "Sacred" is experienced—physically and emotionally—as complete rightness in the moment. The sacred is not reasoned or abstracted, but felt. It is phenomenological or anthropological, rather than theological or medical. Within the sacred, the mystery of life is miraculous. There is no terror, only awe. All paradox and conflict are resolved, or, more precisely, dissolve. In sacred places or sacred moments a person experiences: Being infinitesimal *and* infinite. Being utterly vulnerable *and* unshakably confident. Having inherent meaning despite individual insignificance. The completeness of *this moment*—here and now—within the limitless expanse of all that is, was, and will be.

This is not intoxication in any sense. In fact, it is a deep awareness of the true nature of reality, a sense of being fully, firmly grounded.

Religions teach that experiences of the sacred are always available for those who can access this level of awareness. But for the vast majority of us, the threshold for perception is crossed more readily in places like cathedrals, be they human made, such as Notre Dame, Angkor Wat, the Wailing Wall, or Mecca, or natural cathedrals, such as the Grand Canyon, Himalayan peaks, or an ocean's endless expanse. For me and many of us who are drawn to medicine and nursing, the doors to the sacred are thrown open at times of birth and at times of death.

We live in extraordinary times and face unprecedented challenges. Yet, the era in which we live is merely the latest chapter in the unfolding history of human civilization. Each generation can further weave, and thereby strengthen, or neglect and weaken, the civilized fabric it hands down to the next. The loom is currently ours.

Extraordinary challenges often carry extraordinary opportunities. Caring well for the unprecedented numbers of aged and chronically ill people will require—in fact, *already requires*—decisive social and political actions. We urgently need to get started. While we strive to correct deficiencies in our health care and social systems and alleviate people's suffering, we must aim high. Clinicians, clergy, community service providers, politicians, and civic leaders can collaborate in imagining what healthy last chapters of life look like. Only then can we deliver the best possible care and family support.

Through the influence of our nation's media and culture, by caring well for our frailest and most vulnerable members, Americans can help raise expectations and improve care for many people right now and in the years to come. We can make it clear that the best care possible does not stop with excellent disease treatments; that it includes concern for a person's physical comfort, emotions, and spiritual well-being. In so doing, we can protect the breadth of our human endowment in ways that will be felt long into the future.

We need not—*must not*—allow the difficulties we face, or the seriousness of our efforts, to discourage or dishearten us. Our most effective actions will be motivated by love of one another and performed with joy. The healthiest response to death is to love, honor, and celebrate life.

To life!

Acknowledgments

I am grateful to many people for making it possible to tell the stories within this book.

The generosity of Jack and Dorothy Byrne has enabled our Palliative Care Service at Dartmouth-Hitchcock Medical Center to take root and give the best care we can to many people who are in the midst of the worst time in their lives.

The leadership of Dartmouth-Hitchcock has continued to support our program amid competing priorities and intense financial pressures that pervade American health care in recent years. My department chair, Tom Dodds, has encouraged our team to pursue the goal of extending palliative care to seriously and critically ill patients throughout our health system.

My colleagues, the members of DHMC's Palliative Care Service, inspire me through their own high standards and unspoken commitment to give every patient and family the best care they can. The individuals who comprise this team are: Sharona Sachs, Frances Brokaw, Diane Palac, Lisa Stephens, Peggy Bishop, Marie Bakitas, Margaret Hahn, Linda Piotrowski, Donna Soltura, Patricia Parker,

Briane Pinkson, Wendy Sichel, Yvonne Corbeil, Kim DeVillers, Andrea Maile, and Sandra Knowlton-Soho, as well as our extended family, Deborah Steele, Lisa Harbus, Marv Klassen-Landis, and Rebecca Gottesman. The No One Alone volunteers do so much for patients and families. They expand our team in ways that deepen our services and lift all of our spirits.

Every day, patients and families entrust our team with their care. It is a privilege that bears the weight of responsibility. I am grateful to the many patients and families whose experiences contributed to these chapters.

A number of patients, colleagues, relatives, and friends are named within these pages: Antonia Altomare, Perry Ball, Hervey and Joan Durocher, Marc Ernstoff, John Gemery, Jeanne Goldberg Gider, Edith Glikin, Sandy and Jenny Glikin, Susan Glikin Olan, Stuart Gordon, Hal Manning, Herb Maurer, John Mecchella, Letha Mills, Nancy Nye, Marc Pipas, Greg Ripple, Richard Schramm, Margaret Stephens, Michelle Stuhl, Clare Wilmot, Hope Nye Yeager, Bassim Zaki, and Mickey and Sandy Zimble. I am grateful to them all.

I have not met Jeff Corwin, but I want to say to him, "Thank you very much!" for giving "Sharon" one of the best days of her life.

Gail Ross is my literary agent and friend whose belief in my writing has encouraged me to persist in this avocation. During the long development of this project, Gail and her partner, Howard Yoon, spurred me to explore new ways of making the unvarnished facts of dying and caregiving accessible and compelling.

Kenneth Wapner, my friend and writing colleague, contributed his invaluable creative perspective, and skillful word craft during the first drafts of the proposal. His steadfast affirmation and support fortified my confidence in writing this book.

Behind the scenes, Carol Parks masterfully coordinates my lecturing, consulting, and travel. Her patient ability to organize myriad details enables me to focus on doctoring and writing.

I have been fortunate to have Lucia Watson as my editor. Lucia saw the polished sculpture within the material and helped me to refine the shape and arc of the book. Her keen ear kept my voice in tune, enabling me to speak my mind more clearly.

Yvonne Corbeil, my wife, dearest friend, and closest colleague, has been integral to every phase of this project from its inception as an idea, through the research, interviews, writing, and serial revisions of the manuscript. As with so much else in my life, this book would not have been possible without her.

Notes

INTRODUCTION

3 *where they would want to spend their final days:* Barnato, A. E., D. L. Anthony, J. Skinner, P. M. Gallagher, and E. S. Fisher. "Racial and Ethnic Differences in Preferences for End-of-Life Treatment." *J Gen Intern Med* 24 (6) (June 2009): 695–701.

4 *In a health surveillance study:* Azoulay, E., F. Pochard, N. Kentish-Barnes, et al. "Risk of Post-Traumatic Stress Symptoms in Family Members of Intensive Care Unit Patients." *Am J Respir Crit Care Med* 171 (9) (May 1, 2005): 987–994.

5 *one in five adults is 65 or older: An Ageing World: 2008.* Washington, D.C.: U.S. Census Bureau, July 2009, p. 79. Available at: http://www.census.gov/prod/2009pubs/p95-09-1.pdf (accessed August 2011).

5 *2.1 workers for every beneficiary by 2030:* "The Ghost of Social Security." *Wall Street Journal,* July 12, 2000, p. A26.

6 *Institute of Medicine:* Institute of Medicine Committee on Care at the End of Life. *Approaching Death: Improving Care at the End of Life.* Washington, D.C.: National Academy Press, 1997. Institute of Medicine Committee on Cancer Survivorship and National Research Council. *From Cancer Patient to Cancer Survivor: Lost in Transition.* Washington, D.C.: National Academy Press, 2001. Institute of Medicine Committee on Quality of Health Care in America. *Crossing the Quality Chasm: A New Health System for the 21st Century.* Washington, D.C.: National Academy Press, 2005.

7 *"a culture of death":* "How the Culture of Death Was Brought to American Medicine." Available at: http://www.lifetree.org/timeline/EOLchronology.pdf (accessed August 2011).

10 *the way Americans die remains a national disgrace:* Half of all Medicare beneficiaries spent more than $3,103 out of pocket on health care in 2006. The oldest and poorest beneficiaries spent about a quarter of their income on health care. Nonnemaker, L., and S.-A. Sinclair. *Medicare Beneficiaries' Out-of-Pocket Spending for Health Care.*

Washington, D.C: AARP Public Policy Institute, January 2011. Available at: http://
assets.aarp.org/rgcenter/ppi/health-care/ i48-oop.pdf (accessed August 2011).

1. THE BEST CARE POSSIBLE

16 *There is roughly a 75 percent chance of getting through neoadjuvant treatment and having*
    surgery: Greer, S. E., J. M. Pipas, J. E. Sutton, et al. "Effect of Neoadjuvant Therapy
    on Local Recurrence After Resection of Pancreatic Adenocarcinoma." *J Am Coll*
    Surg 206 (3) (March 2008): 451–457. Facts related to the incidence and treatment
    of pancreatic cancer can be found at: http://www.cancer.net/patient/Cancer+
    Types/Pancreatic+Cancer (accessed August 2011).

24 *modern doctors are taught to view sick patients through a lens that primarily sees their medical*
    problems: Weed, L. L. "The Problem-Oriented Record as a Basic Tool in Medical
    Education, Patient Care and Clinical Research." *Ann Clin Res* 3 (3) (June 1971):
    131–134. Weed, L. "The Problem-Oriented Record—Its Organizing Principles and
    Its Structure." *League Exch* (103) (1975): 3–6.

2. BETWEEN SCYLLA AND CHARYBDIS

44 *best practices of this sort usually consume a lot less time and resources:* Lilly, C. M., D. L. De
    Meo, L. A. Sonna, et al. "An Intensive Communication Intervention for the Criti-
    cally Ill." *Am J Med* 109 (6) (October 15, 2000): 469–475. Lilly, C. M., L. A. Sonna,
    K. J. Haley, and A. F. Massaro. "Intensive Communication: Four-Year Follow-up from
    a Clinical Practice Study." *Crit Care Med* 31 (5 Suppl.) (May 2003): S394–S399. Nel-
    son, J. E., K. A. Puntillo, et al. "In Their Own Words: Patients and Families Define
    High-Quality Palliative Care in the Intensive Care Unit." *Crit Care Med* (3) (2010):
    808–818.

45 *Advance directives—a living will or a durable power of attorney for health care:* Parker,
    K. *Coping With End-of-Life Decisions: Few Have Living Wills.* Pew Research Cen-
    ter, August 20, 2009. Available at: http://pewresearch.org/pubs/1320/opinion-
    end-of-life-care-right-to-die-living-will.pdf (accessed August 2011). Agency for
    Healthcare Research and Quality Advance Care Planning. "Preferences for Care at
    the End of Life." *Research in Action* 12 (March 2003). Available at: http://www.ahrq
    .gov/research/endliferia/endria.pdf (accessed August 2011). Span, P. "Why Do We
    Avoid Advance Directives?" *New York Times*, April 20, 2009.

49 *There are 3,228 hospitals with ICUs and a total of over 67,000 ICU beds in our country,*
    and many are occupied by people who have been critically ill for weeks on end: Carr, B. G.,
    D. K. Addyson, and J. M. Kahn. "Variation in Critical Care Beds per Capita
    in the U.S.: Implications for Pandemic and Disaster Planning." *JAMA* 303 (14)
    (April 14, 2010): 1371–1372. Nelson. J. E., C. E. Cox, A. A. Hope, and S. S. Carson.
    "Chronic Critical Illness." *Am J Respir Crit Care Med* 182 (4) (August 15, 2010):
    446–454. Nelson, J. E., D. E. Meier, A. Litke, D. A. Natale, R. E. Siegel, and
    R. S. Morrison. "The Symptom Burden of Chronic Critical Illness." *Crit Care Med*
    32 (7) (July 2004): 1527–1534.

52 *after slowly rewarming him to 37° centigrade (98.6 Fahrenheit), he remains densely coma-*
    tose with no sign of neurological recovery: Cox, C. E., T. Martinu, et al. "Expectations

and Outcomes of Prolonged Mechanical Ventilation." *Crit Care Med* 37 (11) (2009): 2888–2894, quiz 2904.

56 *a chronically critically ill patient in the ICU:* The term "chronically critically ill" was first used by critical care physicians Girard and Raffin in an article in 1985. Girard, K., and T. A. Raffin. "The Chronically Critically Ill: To Save or Let Die?" *Respir Care* 30 (5) (1985): 339–347.

57 *In her book* Refuge: Williams, T. T.. *Refuge: An Unnatural History of Family and Place.* New York: Vintage Books, 1991.

58 *She chose* It's Always Something *for the title of her book about living with cancer:* Radner, G. *It's Always Something.* New York: Simon & Schuster, 1989.

3. BALANCING ACT

73 *advances decisional science and its application in practice:* The materials available through the Foundation for Informed Medical Decision Making, Healthwise, and the Center for Shared Decision Making provide patients and families with relevant information and, whenever possible, evidence-based guides. This is consistent with the process of innovation that C. Christensen, J. Grossman, and J. Hwang discuss in *The Innovator's Prescription.* New York: McGraw-Hill, 2009.

77 *leaving a legacy for his children, grandchildren, and generations to come:* Baines, B. K. "Writing an Ethical Will." *Minn Med* 87 (1) (January 2004): 26–28. Gessert, C. E., B. K. Baines, S. A. Kuross, C. Clark, and I. V. Haller. "Ethical Wills and Suffering in Patients with Cancer: A Pilot Study." *J Palliat Med* 7 (4) (August 2004): 517–526.

90 *Uncertainty underlies much of the stress and anxiety associated with making decisions about medical treatments:* Kars, M. C., M. H. Grypdonck, A. Beishuizen, E. M. Meijer-van den Bergh, and J. J. van Delden. "Factors Influencing Parental Readiness to Let Their Child with Cancer Die." *Pediatr Blood Cancer* 54 (7) (July 1, 2010): 1000–1008. Hebert, R. S., R. Schulz, V. C. Copeland, and R. M. Arnold. "Preparing Family Caregivers for Death and Bereavement: Insights from Caregivers of Terminally Ill Patients." *J Pain Symptom Manage* 37 (1) (January 2009): 3–12.

4. PALLIATIVE CARE

97 *palliative medicine . . . earned status as a subspecialty in September 2006:* Palliative medicine is now an officially accepted subspecialty that can be earned and added to a physician's primary specialty in ten disciplines. The primary specialties of internal medicine, family medicine, surgery, pediatrics, emergency medicine, physical medicine and rehabilitation, anesthesiology, psychiatry and neurology, radiology, and obstetrics and gynecology cosponsored the young discipline's application before the American Board of Medical Specialties. As of August 2011, there were a total of eighty-two active programs offering more than 210 fellowship positions. Seventy-seven programs have been accredited by the Accreditation Council for Graduate Medical Education and five programs have been accredited by the American Osteopathic Association. Some programs include an additional track in research, geriatrics, or public health.

104 *federal law passed in 1981 that established the Medicare benefit for hospice care restricted eligibility:* http://www.medicareadvocacy.org/medicare-info/medicare-hospice-benefit/ (accessed August 2011). The official "Medicare Hospice Benefit" brochure is available at: http://www.medicare.gov/publications/pubs/pdf/02154.pdf (accessed August 2011).

107 *Research now shows that many people live longer with hospice care:* Connor, S. R., B. Pyenson, K. Fitch, C. Spence, and K. Iwasaki. "Comparing Hospice and Nonhospice Patient Survival Among Patients Who Die Within a Three-Year Window." *J Pain Symptom Manage* 33 (3) (March 2007): 238–246.

108 *Convincing evidence of the capacity of palliative care to simultaneously improve quality and extend length of life:* Temel, J. S., J. A. Greer, A. Muzikansky, et al. "Early Palliative Care for Patients with Metastatic Non-Small-Cell Lung Cancer." *N Engl J Med* 363 (8) (August 19, 2010): 733–742. El-Jawahri, A., J. A. Greer, and J. S. Temel. "Does Palliative Care Improve Outcomes for Patients with Incurable Illness? A Review of the Evidence." *J Supp Oncol* 9 (3) (2011): 87–94.

109 *team-based palliative care:* According to a survey by the Center to Advance Palliative Care, 100 percent of AAMC member teaching hospitals reported having a palliative care program; in 2008 over 81 percent of hospitals with more than 300 beds had a palliative care program. Kirch, D. G. "A Word from the President—Embracing the Value of Palliative Medicine." *AAMC Reporter.* June 2011. Available at: https://www.aamc.org/newsroom/reporter/june2011/250904/word.html (accessed August 2011).

112 *diminish post-traumatic stress among family members after a patient has been in the ICU:* Azoulay, E., F. Pochard, N. Kentish-Barnes, et al. "Risk of Post-Traumatic Stress Symptoms in Family Members of Intensive Care Unit Patients." *Am J Respir Crit Care Med* 171 (9) (May 1, 2005): 987–994. Lautrette, A., M. Darmon, B. Megarbane, et al. "A Communication Strategy and Brochure for Relatives of Patients Dying in the ICU." *N Engl J Med* 356 (5) (February 1, 2007): 469–478. Lilly, C. M., L. A. Sonna, K. J. Haley, and A. F. Massaro. "Intensive Communication: Four-Year Follow-up from a Clinical Practice Study." *Crit Care Med* 31 (5 Suppl.) (May 2003): S394–S399. Curtis, J. R., and D. B. White. "Practical Guidance for Evidence-Based ICU Family Conferences." *Chest* 134 (4) (October 2008): 835–843. This article succinctly presents a straightforward approach to family meetings that is supported by evidence.

112 *Dr. Bakitas's research team at Dartmouth-Hitchcock Medical Center reviewed charts of one hundred patients who died in our hospital during 2008:* Bakitas, M., P. Parikh, F. C. Brokaw, et al. "Has There Been Any Progress in Improving the Quality of Hospitalized Death? Replication of a U.S. Chart Audit Study." *BMJ* (in press August 2011).

000 *Studies have shown that a physician's response to the surprise question is a significant prognostic indicator:* Moss, A. H., J. Ganjoo, S. Sharma, et al. "Utility of the 'Surprise' Question to Identify Dialysis Patients with High Mortality." *Clin J Am Soc Nephrol* 3 (5) (September 2008): 1379–1384. Moss, A. H., J. R. Lunney, S. Culp, et al. "Prognostic Significance of the 'Surprise' Question in Cancer Patients." *J Palliat Med* 13 (7) (July 2010): 837–840.

5. MORBIDITY AND MORTALITY

126 *many states' laws grant M&M conferences special protection from being discoverable in civil malpractice litigation:* Griffen, D. F. "The Challenge to Confidentiality in Peer Review." *Bulletin of the American College of Surgeons* 84 (5) (May 1999).

127 *The tradition began in the field of surgery:* Prasad,V. "Reclaiming the Morbidity and Mortality Conference: Between Codman and Kundera." *Med Humanit* 36 (2) (December 2010): 108–111.

146 *the longer a seriously injured or ill person requires a ventilator to breathe:* Unroe, M., J. M. Kahn, S. S. Carson, et al. "One-Year Trajectories of Care and Resource Utilization for Recipients of Prolonged Mechanical Ventilation: A Cohort Study." *Ann Intern Med* 153 (3) (August 3, 2010): 167–175. Cox, C. E., T. Martinu, S. J. Sathy, et al. "Expectations and Outcomes of Prolonged Mechanical Ventilation." *Crit Care Med* 37 (11) (November 2009): 2888–2894; quiz 2904.

6. WHAT ARE DOCTORS FOR?

157 *Most medical schools do not require hospice or palliative care rotations:* Van Aalst-Cohen, E. S., R. Riggs, and I. R. Byock. "Palliative Care in Medical School Curricula: A Survey of U.S. Medical Schools." *J Palliat Med* 11 (9) (November 2008): 1200–1202.

159 *elders without dementia who were in severe pain after surgery had nine times the risk of becoming delirious, compared to patients whose pain was properly treated with morphine:* Morrison, R. S., J. Magaziner, et al. "Relationship Between Pain and Opioid Analgesics on the Development of Delirium Following Hip Fracture." *J Geront. Series A, Biological Sciences and Medical Sciences* 58 (1) (2008): 76–81.

160 *a famous aphorism in medicine:* "To cure sometimes, *to relieve* often, to comfort always." Possible origins of this quotation are discussed in L. M. Payne, *"Guerir quelquefois, soulager souvent, consoler toujours."* *Br Med J* 4 (5570) (October 7, 1967): 47–48.

163 *to ensure they were not suffering as they died:* Quill, T. E., and I. R. Byock. "Responding to Intractable Terminal Suffering: The Role of Terminal Sedation and Voluntary Refusal of Food and Fluids." ACP-ASIM End-of-Life Care Consensus Panel. American College of Physicians–American Society of Internal Medicine. *Ann Intern Med* 132 (5) (March 7, 2000): 408–414.

168 *"a doctor who has never been tempted to kill a patient probably has had limited clinical experience or is not able to empathize with those who suffer":* Twycross, R. G. *Introducing Palliative Care.* Twycross. "Euthanasia: Going Dutch?" *J Royal Soc Med* 89 (2) (February 1996): 61–63.

170 *you take what you need and leave the rest:* Lyric by Robbie Robertson, "The Night They Drove Old Dixie Down." 1969.

172 *It's always too soon, until it's too late:* The expression "It's always too soon, until it's too late" is used by many of us in the field. I learned it from Dr. Lachlan Forrow, a palliative care physician and ethicist at Beth Israel Deaconess and Harvard Medical School. The expression may have originated from Dr. Judith Nelson, a critical care and palliative care physician at New York's Mount Sinai Medical Center, who coined the phrase "It's too early until it's too late."

173 *several sites on the Internet:* Advance Directives are available for download from the following sites: Caring Connections: http://www.caringinfo.org/i4a/pages/index.cfm?pageid=3289 (accessed August 2011); Center for Practical Bioethics: http://practicalbioethics.org/about/model-and-methodology/making-your-wishes-known-for-end-of-life-care/(accessed August 2011); New York Online Access to Health: http://www.noah-health.org/en/rights/endoflife/adforms.html (accessed August 2011).

179 *Doctors can help people identify meaningful things they can still accomplish or achieve:* There are a number of quality of life tools available to assist with this process: Stiel, S., K. Kues, N. Krumm, L. Radbruch, and F. Elsner. "Assessment of Quality of Life in Patients Receiving Palliative Care: Comparison of Measurement Tools and Single Item on Subjective Well-Being." *J Palliat Med* 14 (5) (May 2011): 599–606. Hales, S., C. Zimmermann, and G. Rodin. "The Quality of Dying and Death: A Systematic Review of Measures." *Palliat Med* 24 (2) (March 2010): 127–144. Steinhauser, K. E., E. C. Clipp, H. B. Bosworth, et al. "Measuring Quality of Life at the End of Life: Validation of the QUAL-E." *Palliat Support Care* 2 (1) (March 2004): 3–14. Byock, I. R., and M. P. Merriman. "Measuring Quality of Life for Patients with Terminal Illness: The Missoula-VITAS Quality of Life Index." *Palliat Med* 12 (4) (1998): 231–244. Steele, L. L., B. Mills, et al. "The Quality of Life of Hospice Patients: Patient and Provider Perceptions." *Am J Hosp Palliat Care* 22 (2) (2005): 95–110. Cohen, S. R., B. M. Mount, et al. "The McGill Quality of Life Questionnaire: A Measure of Quality of Life Appropriate for People with Advanced Disease. A Preliminary Study of Validity and Acceptability." *Palliat Med* 9 (3) (1995): 207–219.

7. THE BUSY DAY THAT SHARON DIED

200 *To be of use:* "To Be of Use" from *Circles on the Water* by Marge Piercy, copyright © 1982 by Middlemarch, Inc., used by permission of Alfred A. Knopf, a division of Random House, Inc.

214 *Sharon religiously watched Jeff Corwin's show on Animal Planet:* Jeff Corwin is host of *Animal Planet* on the Discovery Channel and a leading conservationist. More information at: http://animal.discovery.com/fansites/jeffcorwin/jeffcorwin.html (accessed August 2011).

8. FIXING HEALTH CARE

230 *It is one of the reasons that doctors are burning out in unprecedented numbers:* Male doctors are fourteen times more likely to commit suicide than other men, and female doctors are twenty-three times more likely to do so than other women, according to a 2004 analysis in the *American Journal of Psychiatry*. Devi, S. "Doctors in Distress." *Lancet* 377 (9764) (2011): 454–455. Relevant statistics of professional burnout among physicians and an excellent discussion of the causes and potential strategies for preventing and managing stress can be found in Kearney, M. K., R. B. Weininger, et al. "Self-Care of Physicians Caring for Patients at the End of Life: Being Connected . . . a Key to My Survival." *JAMA* 301 (11) (2009): 1155–1164, E1151.

235 *average costs during the last two years of life ranged from $93,842 per patient at UCLA Medical Center in Los Angeles to $53,432 at Mayo Clinic in Minnesota:* Wennberg, J. E., S. Brownlee, E. S. Fisher, J. S. Skinner, and J. N. Weinstein. *An Agenda for Change: Improving Quality and Curbing Health Care Spending.* A report of the Dartmouth Atlas Project, Dartmouth Institute for Health Policy and Clinical Practice, December 2008. Available at: http://www.dartmouthatlas.org/downloads/reports/agenda_for_change.pdf (accessed August 2011).

235 *a nearly fourfold difference in cities that are a car ride apart:* Goodman, D. C., E. S. Fisher, C. H. Chang, N. E. Morden, J. O. Jacobson, K. Murray, and S. Miesfeldt. *Quality of End-of-Life Cancer Care for Medicare Beneficiaries: Regional and Hospital-Specific Analyses.* A report of the Dartmouth Atlas Project, Dartmouth Institute for Health Policy and Clinical Practice, November 2010. Available at: http://www.dartmouthatlas.org/downloads/reports/Cancer_report_11_16_10.pdf (accessed August 2011).

235 *Congress passed the Medicare Hospice Benefit in 1982:* Public Law 97-248, 1982. Scheduled for implementation in 1983. Available at: http://history.nih.gov/research/downloads/PL97-248.pdf (accessed August 2011).

236 *national median length of hospice service ranges from sixteen to twenty days:* More information at: http://www.nhpco.org/i4a/pages/index.cfm?pageid=5994 (accessed August 2011).

236 *Atul Gawande, set out to get a sense of why the regional disparities described in the* Dartmouth Atlas *occurred:* McAllen costs Medicare seven thousand dollars more per person each year than does the average city in America. McAllen, Tex.—$14,946; El Paso, Tex.—$7,504; Rochester, N.Y.—$6,688 (2006 numbers). Gawande, A. "The Cost Conundrum." *New Yorker,* June 1, 2009. Read more at: http://www.newyorker.com/online/blogs/newsdesk/2009/06/atul-gawande-the-cost-conundrum-redux.html#ixzz1CSIPcGfO (accessed August 2011).

237 *It is high time that American doctors take a hard look at the reasons we do what we do:* The Dartmouth Atlas Project findings have been criticized by institutions delivering the highest intensities of medical care. By focusing only on cases in which patients died and looking back at what happened for a fixed period of time before death, the Dartmouth Atlas methodology would not see patients who survived against all odds. There is no evidence that miracle cures occur more often at the highest costs centers compared to places such as Mayo Clinic or Cleveland Clinic with nearly half the costs at the end of life. Nevertheless, from a public health perspective, the basic conclusion stands: more treatment is associated with outcomes—such as dying in a hospital or an ICU, and spending little time at home—that most people do not want.

238 *multicenter study of eight acute-care hospitals with mature Palliative Care Services compared patients served by palliative care to matched controls:* Morrison, R. S., J. D. Penrod, J. B. Cassel, et al. "Cost Savings Associated with U.S. Hospital Palliative Care Consultation Programs." *Arch Intern Med* 168 (16) (September 8, 2008): 1783–1790. See also Morrison, R. S., J. Dietrich, S. Ladwig, et al. "Palliative Care Consultation Teams Cut Hospital Costs for Medicaid Beneficiaries." *Health Affairs* 30 (3) (March 2011): 454–463.

242 *report cards with quality ratings of hospitals, nursing homes, and home health agencies:* These can be found at: http://www.medicare.gov (accessed August 2011).

242 *Veteran's Administration transparently publishes health outcomes:* These can be found at: http://www.hospitalcompare.va.gov (accessed August 2011).

243 *The Patient's Bill of Rights and the American Hospital Association's brochure "The Patient Care Partnership":* Both are available at: http://www.aha.org/aha/issues/Communicating -With-Patients/pt-care-partnership.html (accessed August 2011).

9. IMAGINING A CARE-FULL SOCIETY

255 *over 61 million Americans are engaged in the timeless role of caring for an ill or disabled young or old relative:* Valuing the invaluable: 2011 update. *The Economic Value of Family Caregiving in 2009.* AARP Public Policy Institute, July 2011. From the report: "In 2009, about 42.1 million family caregivers in the U.S. provided care to an adult with limitations in daily activities at any given point in time, and about 61.6 million provided care at some time during the year. The estimated economic value of their unpaid contributions was approximately $450 billion in 2009, up from an estimated $375 billion in 2007. The report also explains the contributions of family caregivers, details the costs and consequences of providing family care, and provides recommendations for policies that better support caregivers." Available at: http://assets .aarp.org/rgcenter/ppi/ltc/fs229-ltc.pdf (accessed August 2011). Important earlier reports on the economics of caregiving include: Arno, P. S., C. Levine, and M. N. Memmott. "The Economic Value of Informal Caregiving." *Health Aff (Millwood)* 18 (2) (March–April 1999): 182–188. Haley, W. E., L. A. LaMonde, B. Han, S. Narramore, and R. Schonwetter. "Family Caregiving in Hospice: Effects on Psychological and Health Functioning Among Spousal Caregivers of Hospice Patients with Lung Cancer or Dementia." *Hosp J* 15 (4) (2001): 1–18. Covinsky, K. E., L. Goldman, E. F. Cook, et al. "The Impact of Serious Illness on Patients' Families. SUPPORT Investigators. Study to Understand Prognoses and Preferences for Outcomes and Risks of Treatment." *JAMA* 272 (23) (December 21, 1994): 1839–1844.

255 *husbands and sons are shouldering about a third of caregiving responsibilities:* Horowitz, A. "Sons and Daughters as Caregivers to Older Parents: Differences in Role Performance and Consequences." *Gerontol* 25 (6) (December 1985): 612–617. This older study is representative of traditional findings of differences in prevalence and intensity of family caregiving between sons and daughters. Recent trends indicate increasing proportion of men among family caregivers. Today, as many as one-third of family caregivers are men. One survey found that 39 percent of caregivers were men. The proportion varied by race: 38 percent among whites, 33 percent blacks, 41 percent Hispanics, 56 percent Asian. *Caregiving in the U.S.* A report by National Alliance for Caregiving and AARP, April 2004. Funded by MetLife Foundation. Available at: http://www.caregiving.org/data/04finalreport.pdf (accessed August 2011). Gandel, C. "Men as Caregivers: Stories and Statistics on the Changing Face of Caregiving." *Caring Today,* June 2010. Available at: http://www.caringto day.com/read-caregiver-stories/men-as-caregivers (accessed August 2011). "Fact Sheet: Selected Caregiver Statistics." Family Caregiving Alliance, National Center on Caregiving. Available at: http://www.caregiver.org/caregiver/jsp/content _node.jsp?nodeid=439 (accessed August 2011).

255 *Caregiving in modern times extracts a toll:* Nearly 10 million adults are caring for aging parents. Many of these caregivers are of the baby boom generation and are aging themselves. The percentage of adult children providing personal care and/or financial assistance to a parent has more than tripled over the past fifteen years. Currently, a quarter of adult children, mainly baby boomers, provide these types of care to a parent. This has serious consequences for their own incomes, careers, and financial well-being. *The MetLife Study of Caregiving Costs to Working Caregivers: Double Jeopardy for Baby Boomers Caring for Their Parents.* June 2011. MetLife Mature Market Institute, National Alliance for Caregiving, Center for Long Term Care Research and Policy at New York Medical College. Available at: http://www.guardianship.org/reports/mmi_caregiving_costs_working_caregiv ers.pdf (accessed August 2011). Haley, W. E., L. A. LaMonde, B. Han, S. Narramore, and R. Schonwetter. "Family Caregiving in Hospice: Effects on Psychological and Health Functioning Among Spousal Caregivers of Hospice Patients with Lung Cancer or Dementia." *Hosp J* 15 (4) (2001): 1–18. Schulz, R., and S. R. Beach. "Caregiving as a Risk Factor for Mortality: The Caregiver Health Effects Study." *JAMA* 282 (1999): 2215–2219. An important prospective study using data from a large health surveillance study found that caregivers of spouses who reported physical or emotional strain from caregiving, experienced a 63 percent higher chance of dying over four years than non-caregivers. Hebert, R. S., R. M. Arnold, and R. Schulz. "Improving Well-Being in Caregivers of Terminally Ill Patients. Making the Case for Patient Suffering as a Focus for Intervention Research." *J Pain Symptom Manage* 34 (5) (November 2007): 539–546.

258 *nurses and social workers serve as case managers or health care advocates:* Rose, J. "Don't Underestimate the Nurse." *Marketplace Money.* November 19, 2010. Read more at: http://marketplace.publicradio.org/display/web/2010/11/19/mm-dont-under estimate-the-nurse/ (accessed August 2011).

258 *the best care for seriously ill patients is also the best care for their caregiving husbands and wives:* Christakis, N. A., and T. J. Iwashyna. "The Health Impact of Health Care on Families: A Matched Cohort Study of Hospice Use by Decedents and Mortality Outcomes in Surviving, Widowed Spouses." *Soc Sci Med* 57 (3) (August 2003): 465–475. Hospice services seems to lessen depression among surviving spouses. One study found short (less than three days) of hospice services was associated with a heightened risk of depression among bereaved spouses. Bradley, E. H., H. Prigerson, M. D. Carlson, E. Cherlin, R. Johnson-Hurzeler, and S. V. Kasl. "Depression Among Surviving Caregivers: Does Length of Hospice Enrollment Matter?" *Am J Psychiatry* 161 (12) (December 2004): 2257–2262.

259 *people also commonly report gaining personal value from caring:* AARP Massachusetts End of Life Survey, August 2005. Available at: http://assets.aarp.org/rgcenter/health/ ma_eol.pdf (accessed August 2011). *Nebraska End of Life Survey Report,* Nebraska Hospice and Palliative Care Partnership, January 2007. Available at: http://www .reclaimtheend.org/pdfs/Nebraska%20Survey%20Report%202007.pdf (accessed August 2011). *Idaho Statewide End-of-Life Survey Report,* 2006. Available at: http:// aging.boisestate.edu/pdf/idendoflifesurvey.pdf (accessed August 2011).

259 *inherent drive to provide care:* Pro-social, caring behaviors can be observed in toddlers. Caring impulses are innate and normal attributes of the human condition. Goleman, D. *Emotional Intelligence.* New York: Bantam, 1995. Goleman, D. *Social Intelligence.* New York: Bantam, 2006. Zahn-Waxler, C., M. Radke-Yarrow, E. Wagner, and M. Chapman. "Development of Concern for Others." *Devel Psychol* 28 (1) (January 1992): 126–136. Zahn-Waxler, C., and M. Radke-Yarrow. "The Origins of Empathic Concern." *Motiv and Emo* 14 (2) (1990): 107–130.

259 *The Careless Society:* McKnight, J. *Community and Its Counterfeits.* New York: Basic Books, 1995.

264 *People love the support and sense of community they derive from PACE:* Satisfaction surveys reveal that PACE services are well received. *Wisconsin Partnership Program and PACE Program 2004 Participant Satisfaction Survey.* Available at: http://www.dhs.wisconsin.gov/WIpartnership/pdf-wpp/Participant%20Satisfaction%20Survey.pdf (accessed August 2011).

265 *Many PACE sites focus on people who are medically impoverished and unable to live independently at home:* According to the National Clearinghouse for Long-term Care Information, the average costs in the U.S. (in 2009) were: $198/day for a semiprivate room in a nursing home and $219/day for a private room in a nursing home, which is roughly equivalent to $80,000 per year. Information is available at: http://www.longtermcare.gov/LTC/Main_Site/Paying_LTC/Costs_Of_Care/Costs_Of_Care.aspx (accessed August 2011).

10. STANDING ON COMMON HIGH GROUND

274 *In Pew surveys:* Strong Public Support for Right to Die: *More Americans Discussing—and Planning—End-of-Life Treatment.* A Pew Research Center report. January 5, 2006. Available at: http://people-press.org/files/legacy-pdf/266.pdf (accessed August 2011). *Coping with End-of-Life Decisions: Few Have Living Wills.* A Pew Research Center report. August 20, 2009. Available at: http://pewresearch.org/pubs/1320/opinion-end-of-life-care-right-to-die-living-will (accessed August 2011).

275 *eight citizen forums throughout New Hampshire:* Byock, I. R., Y. J. Corbeil, and M. E. Goodrich. "Beyond Polarization, Public Preferences Suggest Policy Opportunities to Address Aging, Dying, and Family Caregiving." *Am J Hosp Palliat Care* 26 (3) (June–July 2009): 200–208. Full report available at: http://www.reclaimtheend.org/downloads/CitizenVoicesReport.pdf (accessed August 2011). As part of the Medicare Prescription Drug, Improvement, and Modernization Act of 2003, the U.S. Congress created the Citizens' Health Care Working Group. Recommendations of the group are available at: http://govinfo.library.unt.edu/chc/recommendations/finalrecs.html (accessed August 2011).

277 *less distance than many people drive each year:* U.S. drivers average just over 13,000 miles per year—and truck drivers between 80,000 and 120,000 miles annually (according to Answers.com, July 2011, and Federal Highway Administration, April 2011).

279 *StoryCorps:* StoryCorps is a remarkable project that is weaving stories of everyday people into the fabric of American culture. Read more at: http://www.storycorps.org (accessed August 2011).

280 *formal ethical principle and precept of palliative care holds that the practice of palliative care does not intentionally hasten death:* Vanderpool, H. Y. "The Ethics of Terminal Care." *JAMA* 239 (9) (February 27, 1978): 850–852. Byock, I. "Principles of Palliative Care." In Walsh, T. D. (ed.), *Textbook of Palliative Medicine.* Philadelphia: Saunders Elsevier, 2008, pp. 33–41. *A Pathway for Patients and Families Facing Terminal Disease.* National Hospice Organization Standards and Accreditation Committee, 1997. *Clinical Practice Guidelines for Quality Palliative Care.* National Consensus Project for Palliative Care, 2004. Available at: http://www.nationalconsensusproject. org (accessed August 2011). Last Acts Task Force. "Precepts of Palliative Care." *J Palliat Med* 1 (1998): 109–112. *Palliative Care: Towards Standardized Principles of Practice.* Canadian Palliative Care Association, 1995. *Statement on Palliative Care.* World Health Organization. Available at: http://www.who.int/cancer/palliative/ en/ (accessed August 2011). *Cancer Pain Relief and Palliative Care.* Technical Report Series 804. World Health Organization, 1990.

280 *Joseph Cardinal Bernardin:* "Letter to the Supreme Court," by Joseph Cardinal Bernardin, Archbishop of Chicago, November 7, 1996. In *Chicago Tribune,* November 12, 1996. Despite the hyperpartisan political posturing that surrounded the 2009 health care reform debate, most Christians understand the distinction between letting someone die gently and intentionally ending someone's life.

281 *the preamble to the UN's 1948 Universal Declaration of Human Rights:* United Nations General Assembly, 217 A (III) (December 10, 1948). Available at: http://www .unhcr.org/refworld/docid/3ae6b3712c.html (accessed August 2011).

283 *Karen Ann Quinlan, Elizabeth Bouvia, and Nancy Cruzan:* Quinlan ir. 70 NJ 10 355 A2d 647. 1976. A compelling account of the case of Nancy Cruzan and its meaning for American health care can be found in the book *Long Goodbye: The Deaths of Nancy Cruzan* (Carlsbad, Calif.: Hay House, 2002), written by the Cruzans' attorney, William Colby.

292 *You do not need to leave your room:* Franz Kafka (n.d.). Great-Quotes.com., 15:45:47, http://www.great-quotes.com/quote/174670 (accessed August 2011).

Index